MORE THAN PRETTY

Maaria Mozaffar

How to Live a
Life of Substance
in an Artificial World

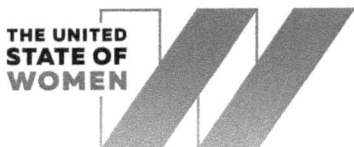

Please purchase additional copies at:
www.YouAreMoreThanPretty.com.

Publishing Consulting by Erika Parsons.

Creative Direction by The Mold Agency.

Copyright © 2017 by Maaria Mozaffar

ISBN: 978-0-692-92033-6

Library of Congress Control Number: 2017949069

Printed in the United States of America.

First Printing: 2017

I dedicate this book to my mother, Yasmeen, the ultimate woman of substance. Thank you for teaching me that the only valuable attribute in a person is character and not to be swayed by the pleasantries of those who don't give it value.

Maaria Mozaffar

Table of Contents

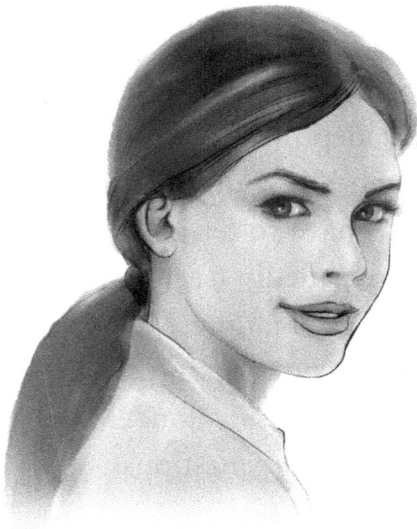

"I see you.
        I understand you."

Introduction

THIS IS NOT A PAT ON THE BACK;
IT IS A PUSH FORWARD

———————

You are here. You cracked open this book, and that means the journey has already begun for you. Perhaps you found this title appealing because you do not feel whole anymore. Or maybe you have grown suspicious of all the superficiality around you and deep down you know you are more. Or you fear for your own little girls or nieces. You fear they will be entering a world that will fill them with insecurity about their looks, their size, their intelligence and their worth. Perhaps you once viewed yourself as a remarkable person of great depth, but somewhere along the way, you convinced yourself that in order to mature, you would have to let go of your ambitions. Perhaps you were actually (secretly) just afraid of challenges and feelings of failure. Whatever the reason that led you here, your picking up this book was no accident. And, you are not alone. Many women struggle to answer the same questions:

- "Where is my life going?"
- "What is my purpose?"
- "Is this all there is?"

There is more to this life than what you have experienced or seen from your individual circumstances. Underneath the pile of negative media messages, toxic interactions, broken promises, washed-up dreams and dysfunctional relationships, there is a far more beautiful landscape of the universe around you and everyone in it. There are champions, living boldly and experiencing joy every day. And they are no different from you. They are filled with optimism, possibility and miracles. This is the world I want to help you discover. This is the world I want you to continue to help build.

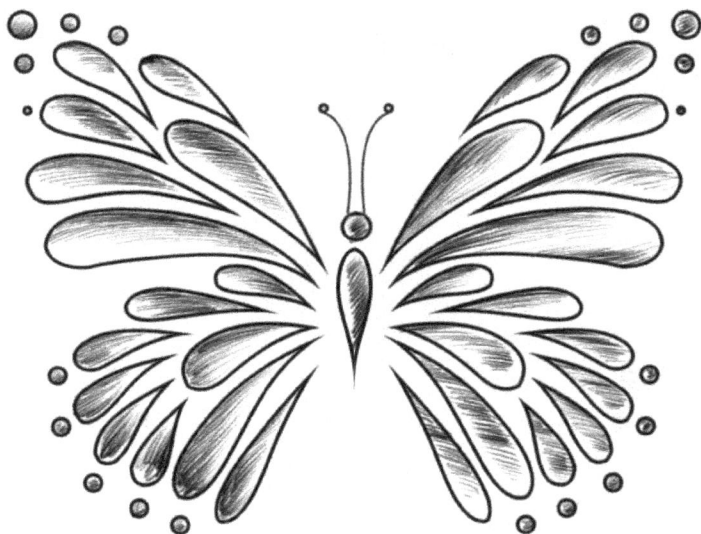

The butterfly effect[1] is defined as one localized moment of change that causes a sequence of grand events. Starting now as you begin this book, I want you to join me in embracing this significant moment in changing the course of your life—your butterfly effect.

---

[1]butterfly effect. (n.d.). Dictionary.com Unabridged. Retrieved March 22, 2017 from Dictionary.com website http://www.dictionary.com/browse/butterfly-effect

Here's what this book is *not*: it is not a tool that gives you a quick fix to joy, confidence, and success. It is not a shortcut to a solution. It won't blame large corporate giants for saddling you with your insecurities or diminishing your self-worth. It doesn't encourage you to focus on the toxicity of others so you can feel righteous in your own skin. This book is not a pat on the back for doing things as usual.

This book *is*, however, the beginning of your next chapter. It's a guide to help you make the next phase of your life the most fulfilling by putting you in the driver's seat. This book will help you dig deeper introspectively. It will force you to examine your interactions, your perceptions of the world and your responsibility to reach your maximum potential. It will outline some of the ways you may unknowingly be contributing to the negative attributes of our world, whether it be poverty, global racism or superficial competition.

You are powerful. You are necessary and your presence among us is deliberate. Thus, you deserve time and attention to sharpen your skills to help you deliver on your purpose with passion.

Women are the foundations of every community. We play the leading role in impacting each coming generation. For such a calling, we need long-term sustainable mental shifts in how we see each other and ourselves. Becoming powerful in your own skin takes work; it takes a resolve to embrace the pain and the joy of life. We need to evaluate how we share ourselves physically, mentally and emotionally so we can be in the driver's seat when facing our circumstances. The path to being extraordinary has no shortcuts and we should not aim for any less. You deserve to reach your greatness. We all have choices. You can take a path with me or follow the crowd and settle for dedicating your time, money and energy to just keeping things at status quo. My suggestion is that you *not* take the easy route. Let's discover this world and your powerful voice in it together. If you take this journey with me, you will:

- Learn how to identify your spiritual compass
- Learn how to build your cocoon
- Learn how to detoxify your life
- Learn how to set your boundaries
- Reaffirm your values
- Discover your purpose
- Connect to a purpose larger than yourself

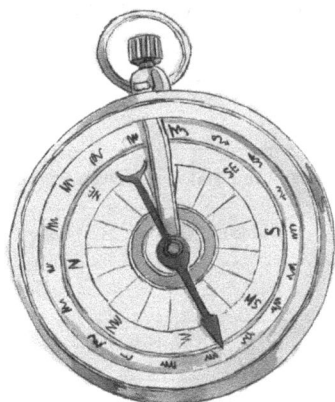

Chapter 1

SPIRITUAL COMPASS

If we want to take a path toward finding our own power, we need to get clear on who or what is guiding us. Humans are all beings searching for something. Have you ever wondered what guides your search or what you are following? Is your top priority meeting your immediate needs like food, sleep, sex, love or sympathy?

We are always operating on two levels:

The First Level (FL) is driven by our body and its immediate needs. The Second Level (SL) is where our cognitive processes reside—a higher level of

FIRST LEVEL		SECOND LEVEL	
Low Stakes	**Signs of Low Stakes**	**High Stakes**	**Signs of High Stakes**
Sex	Passion	Big Picture	Intuition
Money	Jealousy	Working Out	Dicipline
Food	Hunger	Introspection	Gut Feeling
Ego	Competition	Spiritual Contentment	Patience
Short-term Gain	Need to Impress	Long-term Perspective	Red Flag

consciousness. Mostly unseen externally, SL allows us to ponder more deeply and act according to our own moral code. SL guides our actions to help us feel contentment within ourselves and let's us know we are on the right track. SL is also connected to a deeper understanding of our desires. In order to navigate at this level, we all have tools we can tap into every day such as intuition, multi-level analysis of scenarios, and long-term planning.

These two levels get easily confused on a daily basis. Many times we do not see SL as a higher level. We often recognize it as just an addition to our immediate flesh needs without even realizing it. This is where we have to be careful. Our SL "intuitive" level should always guide us to make decisions about our immediate physical needs, not the other way around. I know on paper this seems like common sense. You may be thinking, *Of course, my brain should control what my hands and mouth do.* But trust me, we do not always practice the distinction. Let me share two examples:

1. For the Love of Sugar

Dessert and weight loss is a simple example we all can relate to with lower stakes. You are trying to lose weight, but you are driving by your favorite bakery and you can't resist the urge to stop in and buy a cupcake. You give in and indulge "just this once" to satisfy your craving. No big deal, right? Except that

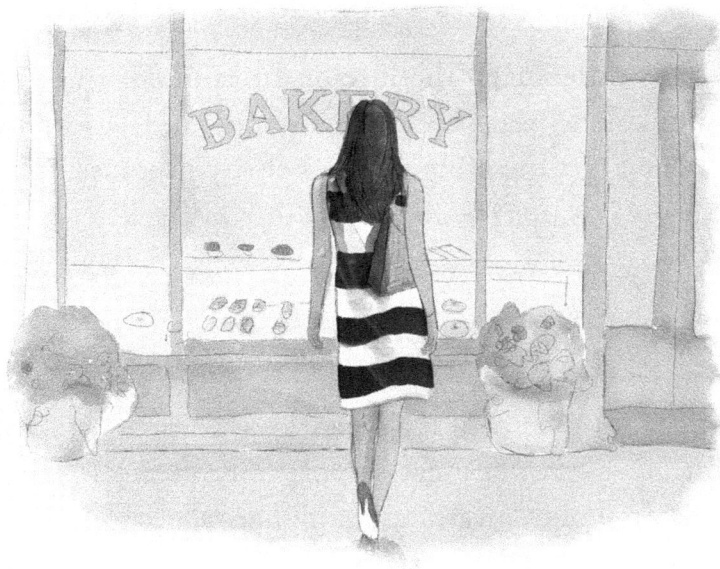

this opens the door to a day of sugar craving. When you are operating at the FL, you would have had the following conversation with yourself that encouraged you to buy the cupcake: "I will work out tomorrow. I really deserve this. It will taste sooo good."

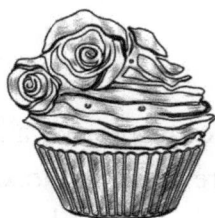

If SL controlled your actions, the internal conversation would go more like this: "A cupcake? Really? This cupcake will just make me want more sugar because that is how my body operates. I will not let my body fall for that immediate satisfaction. This is about self-discipline, not just about saying no to sugar. Not worth it. I'll pass."

See the difference? The lure of the cupcake and not being able to walk away means something more to you in SL. Operating in SL helps you pause. The result is no cupcake and no falling off track.

2. Moving up the Ladder

Career advancement is a scenario with higher stakes. You are offered a great opportunity at work. This position would award you a higher salary and more prestige. But, the role would require you to promote a product you do not support. What would you do? The FL conversation would proceed like this: "This would mean more money and more access to things I can enjoy. I would get more respect from my friends and family. It's only short-term, anyway."

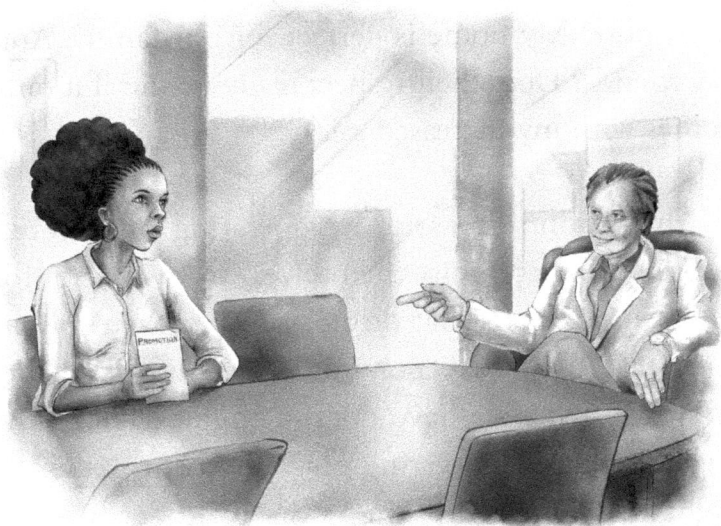

This conversation focuses on your immediate needs, your ego, and your capacity to have material possessions. We get really good at making excellent rationalizations to support FL decisions. The SL conversation goes something like this: "I actually would not ever buy this product. This product is harmful to kids and I know it. If I walk away from this based on the fact that I want to protect kids from product X, I can focus my energy on promoting a product I *would* buy for my kids. They obviously hired me because I understand the industry. Now that I know this product exists, I can create an alternative. It will take time, but it can be my long-term plan. Plus, how much more do I *really need* right now? My home is perfect for our family. And my friends? Does their respect really matter if it only comes with my increased salary?"

In this second scenario, by operating on the FL, people can commit themselves to working for years in positions that do not support their morals or ideals. That may not initially sound like a big deal. Most people have done it, right? Here is the big difference. Operating at your SL to make the right decisions opens the doors to leadership and heightened creativity. It could lead you down a path of entrepreneurship—starting a new company in which you are in control.

Using SL as your guide can enable you to propel you from an ordinary life to an extraordinary one, full of opportunity and purpose. Extraordinary: is that not what we should aim for?

To analyze what level guides you in your small and big decisions is one of the most important foundations of understanding your power in this world. It also forces you to see the significance of *all* your choices, giving you the opportunity to pause, reflect and make better decisions.

Your Guide

Have you ever thought about what allows you to tap into your higher level? It would be disingenuous for me not to share with you that I am a deeply spiritual person of faith, which you probably guessed by the title of this chapter.

I don't want to hide the magic ball from you. No matter how you wish to define Him, Her or It– *there is a higher being.* A higher being that created you, your heart, your mind and this world. This is a foundational reality that a majority of humans believe, search for and have various names for. That internal conversation you are having with yourself—the one that allows you to use your intuition, recognize red flags and see your life in the long term—is aided by the whispers of that higher being. They are whispers to your soul. The question then becomes even more profound and important than what level you are using to make daily decisions. The question becomes *who* or *what* is guiding you? Is it your body or is it what I choose to call God and your Spiritual Compass?

If you are a religious person, that does not mean you are necessarily guided by your Spiritual Compass. In fact, many people use their religious identity and devotion as an external badge, but they are still completely devoid of a spiritual connection. They read, but fail to internalize. They pray, but do not feel. They ask for something in prayer or meditation and promise unconditional acceptance, but secretly fear an outcome they do not want. Many of us are simply not operating at our higher level because we are in a spiritual hibernation.

We are busy running errands, making plans, or complaining of not having any. We are taking care of everyone, criticizing our failures and working hard at trying to be the best. We are awake but somehow asleep at the same time, and that is why we are led to make decisions from our FL. I wanted to start this book by discussing Spiritual Compasses because I was in a spiritual hibernation, as well. It was not until I woke up from it that I was able to operate at a higher level of thinking. And, then everything changed. It is what the Jews interpret the word "Seek" to be in the Old Testament, what the Greeks called "Zeteo," and what the Muslims call "Taqwa" or "God Consciousness." Having this connection in your daily life is the first step in becoming powerful."[2]

I describe it as a gradual shift of my personal compass from the first superficial level to the second higher level. It all started with the birth of my daughter, almost six years ago. The joy and the love I felt was overwhelming. It was then that I came to realize the miracle of a spiritual source I could not comprehend.

I started analyzing the other miracles—personal and professional—that had happened earlier in my life that had gone unnoticed. I had taken success for granted and it made me numb to everyday miracles and opportunities for growth around me. Once I finally woke up, my leanings and interests slowly began to evolve.

I started to appreciate nature at a deeper level. I craved meditative silence. Deep, insightful conversations

---

[2]https://www.skipmoen.com/2012/01/god-consciousness/

excited me. I started to think about how every action I took mattered for the course of my life and for others around me in more significant ways.

I became even better at being present and made it a goal. Wherever I was, I was there in my entirety. This resulted in more inspiration, more joy. And because I slowed down, I was able to use precision in my work, making me much more productive. This insight provided me both with appreciation and disappointment.

> *Faith is my lifeline. I don't believe that my birth was an accident, nor do I believe that my pain was an accident. I try to take every single thing—good or bad— in stride and use it as fuel to leave this world better than I came into it.*
>
> Donnie Smith

I understood what my relationships really meant, whether they aided my spiritual awakening or took me away from it. I realized there was a greater force carrying me through my life the whole time— something bigger than me that was providing me with this ambition and passion. No matter how much I knew this intellectually, it did not become real until I allowed myself to internalize it fully. Once I did, I realized I was responsible for using my actions and decisions wisely no matter how small they may seem initially.

I recently interviewed Donnie Smith, the executive director of Donda's House, Inc., a nonprofit organization co-founded by Kanye West and Che "Rhymefest" Smith. Their mission is to provide access to premium arts instruction to youth, to inspire, challenge and produce tomorrow's problem solvers. Donnie had this to say: "Faith is my lifeline. I don't believe that my birth was an accident, nor do I believe that my pain was an accident. I try to take every single thing—good or bad—in stride and use it as fuel to leave this world better than I came into it."

As we end this chapter, I hope you learn to appreciate the distinction between your first and second level of being. I hope you recognize that by taking this journey to authentic empowerment for yourself, you are guided by a deliberate plan by a higher being. Once we recognize these two important notions, we are ready to launch. So, let's go!

" Value integrity and you will find your way to your power. "

Maaria Mozaffar

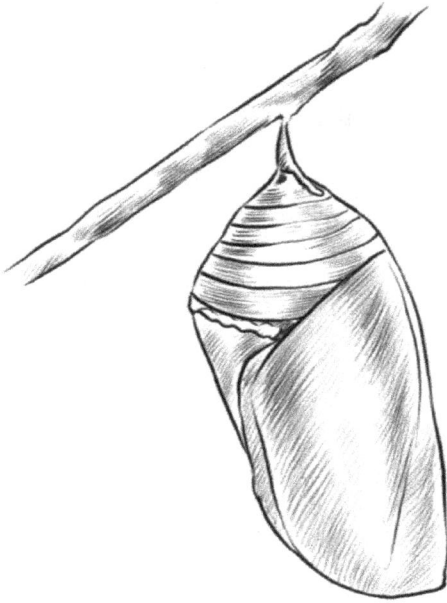

Chapter 2
BABY STEPS TOWARDS A COCOON

Before a butterfly becomes the strong and beautiful version of its complete self, it is encased in a cocoon. Entomologists describe the process as the fifth stage of development, known as the *pupa*. In this stage, which lasts 10 to 14 days, the outer shell, the *chrysalis*, forms. Most people think this stage is a resting phase, but experts say this is where the most crucial development occurs, and the caterpillar actually becomes a full adult.

In order to grow, the butterfly isolates itself from external factors to work on its development. There is a lot we can learn from this process. What if we were able to retreat from our external life in order to develop ourselves?

How Would That Even Happen?

Well, the most important question to ask is *why* we need to take a timeout. I will give you two arguments to encourage the retreat:

    1. We are continually evolving beings.
    2. We are in charge of a coming generation.

Continually Evolving
Like the butterfly, we are constantly developing and falling in and out of life stages. Sometimes these stages are thrust upon us and we are thrown like Dorothy into the tornado. Most of the time, we are happy if we make it to the ground without a house falling on top of us.

Women have obligations relating to college, marriage, motherhood, promotions, elder care, home care, and more. All these stages come with a required set of skills that most women learn to master as the circumstances arise. Sometimes these skill sets are acquired at the cost of our physical and emotional health.

Over the last five years, there has been a sharp rise in anxiety medication use among young adult women. You—with your daily routine of juggling endless to-do lists, short-term and long-term checklists and grocery lists—are not living in a vacuum. You are not alone. There is a ripple effect that is causing a Richter scale needle to constantly shift.

We are all going, day after day, hoping that needle stays at a safe place in each of our 24 hours. Just think about any academic stage of your life. You were expected to study and take tests. If you studied and remained focused, you passed the tests. If you were overwhelmed with confusing concepts in any academic subject, you received a poor grade.

We should look at our life stages the same way. For our practical life, those poor grades come in the form of health problems, stress and more. Since many of us may be in charge of the routines and needs of others, self-neglect can easily happen due to an overwhelmingly long list of items on our checklists. Are not the stakes in our practical life just as high or higher?

The Next Generation

We are also role models to a coming generation. Whether as parents, teachers or caretakers, we have opportunities to model how to be successful and manage stress and others' expectations for the younger generation. If we are not equipped with the right tools, what can we offer those looking to us for guidance? If you are a mother or have had a relationship with your mother, you know full well the impact a mother has on her child. The amount of time she spends with her children gives her endless opportunities to be an example of how to live daily and maximize potential. Among adults, having a "can do" outlook and being an example of productivity can have a ripple effect on your peers and family.

None of this analysis and enlightenment can have any impact unless we are willing to change. In order to implement a change, we need to take a timeout and retreat for ourselves.

How Would That Retreat Look?

For the average woman, it is very difficult to make time for herself. I am not asking you to make time for a three-day retreat and leave your obligations aside. For now, as we begin this process, I am asking you to just take small doable steps called "Checking in" to reserve time for you to grow. Here are some baby steps to building your cocoon. (We will go into greater detail later in the book.)

Morning Check-In

Three mornings a week—let's say Monday, Wednesday and Friday— set your alarm 10 minutes earlier than you normally would and call it "Check-in." In this early hour, splash cold water on your face. Cold water is like a jolt of caffeine in the morning. Keep a pen and paper at your bedside and write your goals for the day during check-in. Note, I did not say *tasks*. The term "task" is daunting, like a chore we would like to avoid, but a *goal* gives you choice and control.

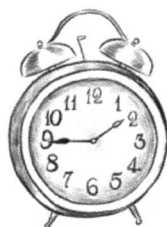

Afternoon Check-In

Around lunchtime, do a 10-minute "Progress Check-in" to review how your day is going. Look at your goal list and make a note of how you are doing, and then adjust where necessary. These goals

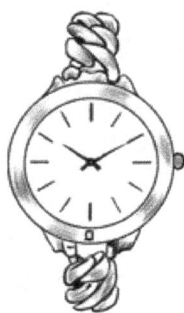

can be professional or personal. After this moment, do not look at your check-in list again until bedtime. The idea is not to stress you out with checklists, but to give you time to process how the day is going. You have checked in twice; move on.

Evening Check-In

In the evening when you have completed your day, take 10 more minutes to look at your list. You should be able to easily see the goals you've achieved for the day and the ones you've moved closer to. It's time to take one more step.

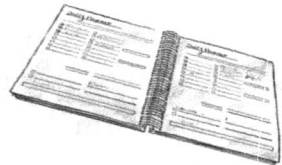

Now, look at each goal and attach an emotion to it. Did it make you feel anxious, sad, happy, or nervous? This is a very important step at the end of the day. Emotions are there to show us how our circumstances are affecting us. Our gut feeling and intuition come into play here.

Being cognizant of these emotions allows that space for you to hear the whispers of your soul. You are being guided every day. Taking the time to plan and analyze that guidance three times a week makes you more aware of your feelings, and gives you little hints as to what you should do next.

As you look through your goal list for the day, and the emotions next to them, pay attention to the emotions that caused you discomfort. Notice, I did not use the phrase "negative feelings." All feelings, even the uncomfortable ones, have a role in your life that serves a purpose. Lean into them and think about how you can make slight changes that evolve those feelings into comfortable ones.

Now, take a few minutes to think about your interactions during the day. If you believe your Spiritual Compass is guiding you, you know that everyone who passed you was a deliberate incident. You'll want to maximize the goodness in every interaction that comes your way, now and in the future. Give yourself a few minutes to think about what you could have done to make the interactions better for both parties. If they were difficult interactions, be in the driver's seat and hold yourself accountable.

Now throw the goal list in the trash. Tomorrow is a new day. These short check-ins are simple steps to help you build your cocoon. They get you accustomed to reserving small amounts of time for yourself to confront your feelings, set goals and gain perspective as a daily practice. You can also combine check-ins with your to-do list, so it doesn't seem so daunting. We would all love to have a personal life coach with us

> *It's important to understand what your underlying emotional issues are that would have you stay in a negative situation. If you don't work through the root cause, you will only recreate the situation again. Once you have this self-awareness, this is when you can make the smart choices.*
>
> *Ariella Ford*

all the time, telling us when to check in and become introspective. For the majority of us, having one is not a option, but this little check in exercise helps us coach ourselves. It allows us talk through and process our feelings, recall our day and develop a different game plan if necessary.

Arielle Ford is a nationally recognized publicist, author, founding member of the Spiritual Cinema Club, and co-producer of Deepak Chopra's *Happiness Prescription*. When I asked her about therapy and coaching, this was her response: "I am a big believer in both. It's important to understand what your underlying emotional issues are that would have you stay in a negative situation. If you don't work through the root cause, you will only re-create the situation. Once you have this self-awareness, this is when you can make the smart choices."

The process of checking in will become automatic for you over time and it will create a habit of emotional self-awareness even if at a small level at first. I recognize that this is a not a huge isolated cocoon. This is why I titled the chapter, "Baby Steps Towards a Cocoon," because to make this book the most useful to you, you will need a little time every day to understand it, reflect on it and apply it. If we can get you in the habit of slowing down every day a little bit for your thoughts, we are closer to getting you to your power.

REMEMBER YOUR DAILY CHECK-INS

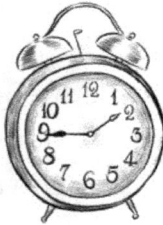

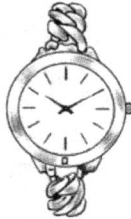

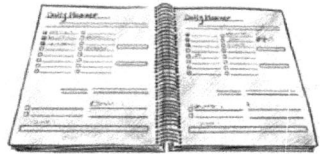

❝ *Let go of unnecessary activities that are not making you happy.* **❞**

Maaria Mozaffar

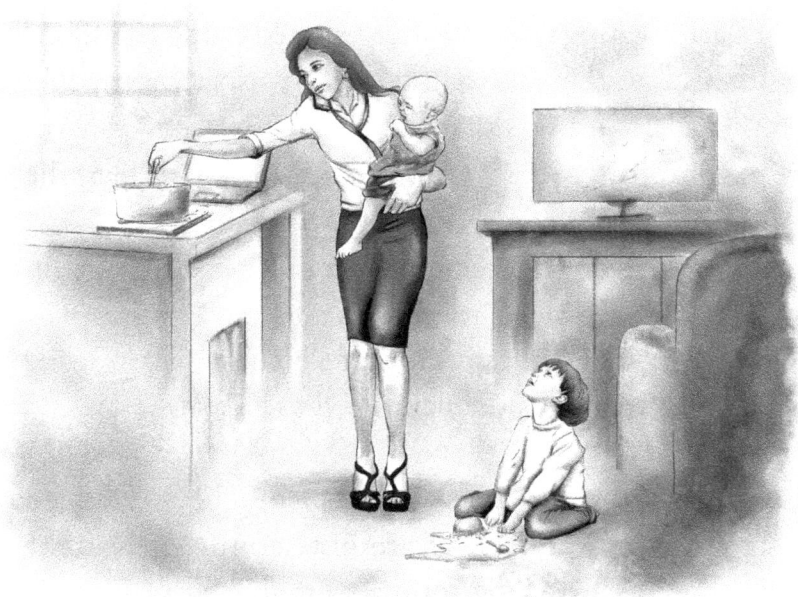

Chapter 3
LET'S DETOX

A detox is a removal of toxins from a functioning system. I have had every combination of kale, spinach, and broccoli imaginable. On the days that I dabble on the dark side of refined sugar, processed carbs, and fatty oils, I always follow with a 24-hour compensation diet with nutrient-rich foods, which include the ABCs of getting back on track: apples, beets, and carrots.

I started eating this way after I started doing triathlons in order to remain healthy in every aspect of my life. What I found was that the things I was choosing to put into my mouth were not serving my body. The toxins were slowing down the functionality of my natural systems, causing my physical state to remain stagnant. We need to continually move forward—emotionally, physically and intellectually; any outside factors keeping us stagnant need to exit stage left.

We need a detox in all areas of our life. We need to let go of things that are not serving us well, or at the very least, learn how to manage our present reality so we can better distinguish between our assets and liabilities.

The Busy Bee

"I know you are busy. So are the bees. But what are you busy doing?"

I don't recall when I first heard this question. But now that I am pulled between personal and professional obligations, I understand why it's such an important one.

“ ...it is imperative that we assess the value of various organizations, activities and events to determine how they fit into God's plans and purpose for our lives. This should be done regularly to remove any spiritual and organizational clutter. ”

Tanesha Pittman

In her article, "Busy is the New Sick," Dr. Susan Koven, an internal medicine physician stated: "In the past few years, I've observed an epidemic of sorts: patient after patient suffering from the same condition. The symptoms of this condition include fatigue, irritability, insomnia, anxiety, headaches, heartburn, bowel disturbances, back pain, and weight gain. There are no blood tests or X-rays diagnostic of this condition, and yet it's easy to recognize. The condition is excessive busyness. It's one with which, as a fellow sufferer, I empathize especially."

I had the opportunity to speak with Tanesha Pittman, Executive Director of the Women's Institute for Global Leadership at Benedictine University Moser College of Adult and Professional Studies. I asked her what advice she has for women who are having a challenging time balancing the important things in life. This is what she said: "I would encourage other women to evaluate how their time is spent. A strategy I use is being more intentional about my commitments or even limited involvement in activities/organizations, etc. Also it is imperative that we assess the value of various organizations, activities and events to determine how they fit into God's plans and purpose for our lives. This should be done regularly to remove any spiritual and organizational clutter."

How many of us are leading lives that are overcommitted, and participating in insincere friendships? It is time to clean up and declutter our homes and our lives. It is time to organize our personal lives, bring sincerity to our relationships and identify our attachment to unnecessary materialistic indulges. We need to learn to manage the ABCs. This means coming up with a game plan to attack the nerve center to uncover why these toxins enter our lives. Here are the three steps we need to follow:

The ABCs of Getting Rid of Life Toxins

1. Assess the WHY. Why do you need the activity or indulgence that is taking your attention and time? If you cannot come up with a reason that helps you move away from remaining stagnant, it's time to decide if this activity—this indulgence—is worth your time.

2. Build boundaries. Set limits on how deeply entrenched you will become while participating in these activities.

3. Calculate the intrinsic value of each activity or indulgence in your life.

Our ultimate catalyst to wanting change is joy. If an activity does not bring you joy, it is an unnecessary drain on your positive energy. Now, let's start with the most dominant new force in our daily lives, social media.

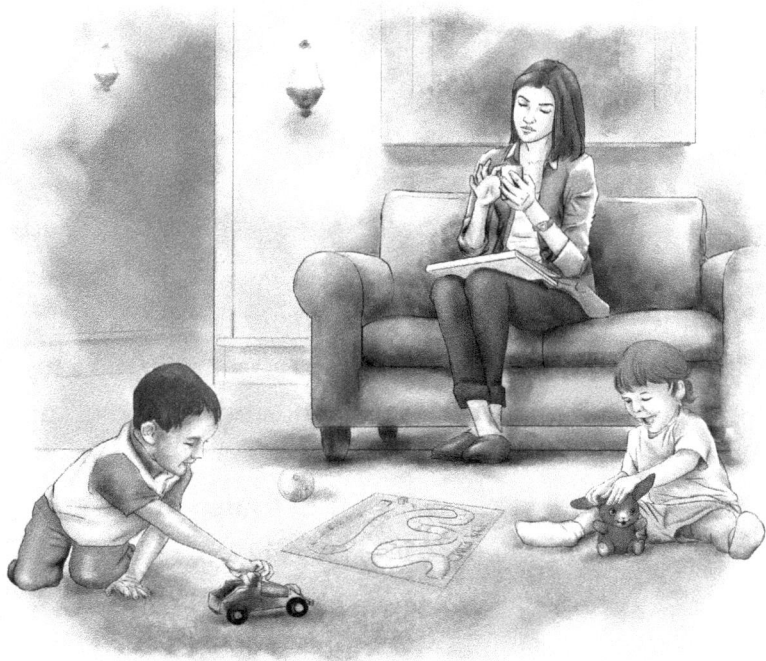

Chapter 4

SOCIAL ANXIETY MEDIA

───────

Social media has impacted all areas of our lives. The new normal has totally changed for the current generation of young adult women. We are experiencing adulthood in a time when everything is rated by the number of likes we receive by our peers. Our private information is public, and the distinctions between private and public are blurred, at best. We cannot pretend that these circumstances have not deeply impacted how we perceive even our most intimate moments. The way we process information and form opinions on current global events is manipulated by the algorithms of our newsfeeds. Even how we plan our social calendar and manage our relationships have dramatically become dependent on technology. Social media makes it easier to schedule and manage our days through platforms like Facebook and Twitter. Communities are making global connections and individuals are finding their long lost friends. Politics, political leaders, and global conflicts are getting exposure in real time.

> *We often think we need to respond instantly to the outside world or fear we are going to miss something if our phone is off, but in reality, being tied to our device causes us to miss the most important moments going on right under our nose.*
>
> *Rachel Stafford*

But the cons of social media, if not managed well, are costing us heavily in our personal lives. We are losing authenticity in our experiences and relationships, which is robbing us of the real intense joys that come from living life.

I had a chance to interview, Rachel Stafford, author of NY Times bestselling book, *Hands Free Mama*. This is her take on social media: "While our devices enable us to virtually work and connect to the Internet anywhere anytime, this availability makes it difficult to draw boundaries between technology and life."

Stafford continues, "We often think we need to respond instantly to the outside world or fear we are going to miss something if our phone is off, but in reality, being tied to our device causes us to miss the most important moments going on right under our nose. I believe that The Hands Free Revolution is resonating with so many people because we are yearning to protect our time, attention, and relationships. Technology has become so invasive and so consuming. People want to know how to let go and simply be in the moment that is their life."

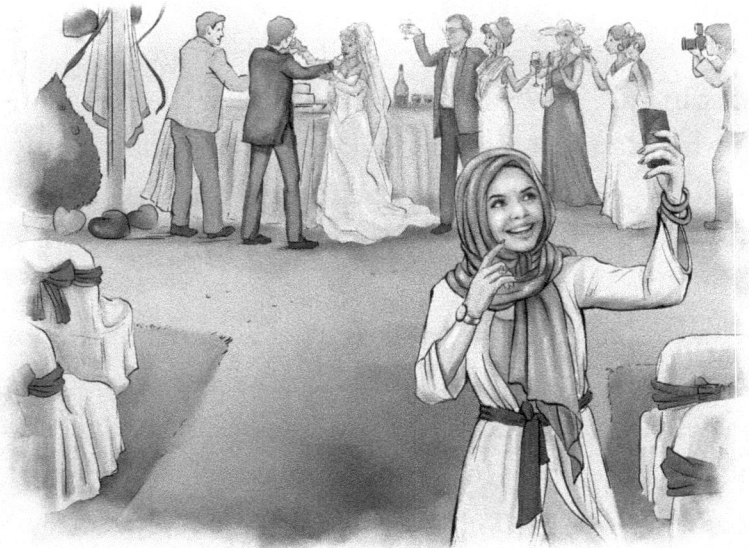

The Selfie

After all, it is just a face. Your face.

The American Psychological Association has recognized the selfie as an emotional, mental sickness. It seems the more people are taking selfies to show the world what they look like while participating in an activity or experience, the more they get addicted to the behavior. They no longer want to share an experience with people, but rather they want to show people what they looked like during the experience. Because after all, what matters most is what they looked like when they took a long, beautiful kayak ride on the Potomac River, right?

This practice alone places a narcissistic need to make every experience we participate in about us. Instead of taking the time to breathe in the fresh air or notice the glimmer of sunshine on the water, our thoughts automatically go to "What angle can we take this selfie from?" We have all done it. We minimize the impact an experience can have on our lives by focusing on ourselves in the moment. This is so harmful because it transforms genuine experience into a self-facing mirror.

That is what the selfie is, in essence, all about. We are obsessed with our face and we want the world to be obsessed with our face, as well. But, here is the news alert: *We are more than our face!*

We are more than our eyes, the shape of our nose and the curves of our jawline. We have a functioning body that helps us accomplish amazing things like giving birth, running marathons, and doing cartwheels. We have a brain that creates our words and ideas, and our contributions to society, and the personal lives of our loved ones. Shouldn't we put effort into developing *all* of the wonderful parts of our mind and body? Here is the second news alert: *Not all faces are created equal.*

This is just the truth. Every cosmetic empire knows that women around the world focus a majority of their time and money trying to deny this truth. With the obsession of Kim Kardashian's skill of contouring, we have further used the selfie to try to make our faces look the same.

Our Creator created various shades, shapes and features. Our obsession with our face, posing like other people and contouring like other people to have a good selfie only reaffirms that we do not find the diversity of our faces beautiful. We have lost the ability to decide the definition of beauty of the face by using our own preferences and faculties.

Notice that I stated *not all faces are created equal,* vs. that all faces are not created the same. And I say this deliberately because we must understand that the consumer-driven industries—cosmetics and fashion—have already chosen for us what is deemed beautiful and some of our faces are just not it. And we will take selfie after selfie, with filter after filter, to fit into a mold that others, specifically corporate boardrooms studying consumer trends, have defined as the ideal. Unless such corporations are paying you, why would you try to become their product or marketing tool? In a nutshell, we have chosen vanity over life experiences.

For the younger, coming-of-age demographic of women, the selfie has a dark side. For impressionable age groups, a lot of emphasis is placed on the face and how many "likes" a selfie receives. Also, how many more "likes" did a friend's selfie receive? These all seem like harmless dynamics, but for a young girl in a society where her self-esteem is always attacked through the media and pop culture messages, the ramifications of putting so much emphasis on your God-given features (which you had no part in achieving) is a self-destructive path.

There is a corporate definition of beauty that these girls are being fed. And their own physical face will change, alter and age and will eventually not fit with the ideal of beauty at some point. "Wearing makeup to enhance one's appearance is normal in our society and often a right of passage for young women," said renowned body image expert, Adrienne Ressler, from the Renfrew Center Foundation. "There is concern, however, when makeup no longer becomes a tool for enhancement but, rather, a security blanket that conceals negative feelings about one's self-image and self-esteem. For many individuals, these feelings may set the stage for addictions or patterns of disordered eating to develop."

Artificial "Perfect" Moments

Social media is a self-promoting public relations firm. Through social media, individuals can hand-pick their best profile pictures, or showcase their perfect marriage, perfect children, thriving career, beautiful home, amazing culinary skills, and table-setting talents. Social media allows people to easily convince everybody that they have a thriving social life complete with a multitude of invitations and busy engagements.

In a lot of ways, setting up a social media profile with pictures and events is much like running a successful political campaign. Anyone who shows that she is liked and wanted will convince others to believe her and like a domino effect, her goal will become a reality. The problem is, of course, that our lives are not political campaigns, and the depths of our experiences are more than perfectly posed photographs. There are two fundamental issues that arise from our obsession with creating shareable picture moments:

1. We internally create a need to have validation from others on the "success" of our lives.

2. We put effort into creating a perfect picture moment in every experience rather than putting effort into making the *experience* picture-worthy.

The effect this practice has on other women sets up an unwinnable competition to have the same success in their lives. In order to attain inclusion in this category, they try to duplicate the same string of artificial images for themselves, creating a vicious cycle yielding no long-term *actual* success for their lives. Let's flesh this out a little bit.

The "Like" Contest

Many of us fall into this trap without even knowing it. It's analogous to selfies robbing us of sensing the actual joy of experiences. Do you remember why we took pictures and how we enjoyed them before social media?

We took pictures to capture memories. In fact, while taking the picture, we would say things in our minds like, "He will love this when he looks back at this time," or, "I am definitely going to show her this when she grows up."

We used to save pictures in a special, safe place, and then dig them up later to flip through albums when we missed someone. What do you say when you take a picture now?

"I can't wait to share this."

This is one of the things we may say out loud. But, let's be honest and think about the things we say internally:

"If I share this, we will look like a magazine cover of the picture-perfect family."

"If I share this, people will see how awesome our marriage is."

"If I share this, people will see how talented I am or how beautiful the decorations looked."

"If I share this, people will see how many friends I have."

"If I share this, people will see that I can afford expensive things."

You may not even say the whole sentence in your mind; it could just be a fragment of thoughts you have while you are looking at the images on your phone or camera. Do you notice the difference between the thoughts we had before the advent of social media and what we have now?

All the thoughts we have regarding pictures now have to do with *other people*. That is where the need for validation creeps in without our even inviting it. It is almost as if we don't consider certain areas of our life a success until we hear again and again from others that they agree. Of course, this comes in the form of "likes," or comments that accentuate the praise to such high degrees that even normal compliments such as "Sweet" or "Pretty" fall short of expected validation. Instead, we get accustomed to seeing and using highly exaggerated phrases on other people's picture images:

"So amazing! You are so talented!"

"What an incredible mother!"

"Absolute stunning!"

"The most lovely couple, inside and out!"

These are statements I am sure we have all seen on our social media pages. Is this how normal people talk? There is a disconnect between the compliments and the value of these compliments themselves. The need for outlandish feedback on our images then develops as a baseline expectation for responses to all our experiences. The result is that we end up minimizing what we actually think about our lives. Instead, we replace it with what others think about our families, our successes and us.

Validation from Others Results in Less Self-Assurance

Studies have shown in the corporate setting, women are much more likely to back away from asking for a promotion and initiating a challenging project, versus men. Most of the time, women feel they are not qualified. They have more to do and more to prove before feeling they are validated to take the next step in their career. The way they make these assessments about themselves is based on their progress review—the things said about them by their peers and superiors. It is almost as if the value they place on how others validate their abilities holds them back from moving forward to grow and enhance their professional portfolio.

The same need for validation is creeping into the personal, family and home life for women that will, in the long-run, start holding them back from moving forward to learn and mature as full adults. Even the most personal experiences such as rearing young children, preparing a feast for their family, or spending family time on the weekend are up for display and an auction block for the highest number of likes. If the images yield high praise, we have achieved success while simultaneously devaluing our own opinion of our personal successes. This creates a space for us to never trust our own judgment. This can actually hold us back from taking a leap on making life-changing decisions:

"Should I have another child?
Look at her, she makes it seem so easy."

"Should I go back to work?
Look at how she balances it;
I would never be able to make it work like her."

"Should I marry him? Look at her husband.
He is more successful and better looking.
Does my fiancé measure up?"

The truth is, we allow the validation of others to steer us into accepting mediocre accomplishments as huge feats. Whether the comments are good or bad, by posting various images of our lives with a hidden intent to show perfection, we allow the validation shown to us by others to have a role in how we feel about ourselves. What makes this situation even more damaging is that we are giving power over ourselves to people who have no real stake in our lives.

We put all our effort into creating the perfect picture of a moment, instead of the memorable experience.

We enhance our photos and place our children and ourselves in perfect poses, on birthdays, anniversaries, and vacations. With the pressure on social media to have an event, invite people and then post pictures of everyone having fun, we tend to place a lot of thought on what to post and share from our life's most precious moments.

The purpose of taking photos has changed from what it was even just 20 years ago. Pictures of our personal, memorable moments allow us to see our grandparents and our parents at a young age on birthdays and anniversary celebrations. We are able to feel the joy and love from a special time because they took the time to take pictures and keep them in organized albums and little picture books. They took them for themselves and future generations and we treasure them.

The original purpose of photos was to keep a special moment in time that can be revisited. Now we have added a new purpose: to share them with hundreds of friends on social media. This changes the game quite a bit. It affects the intent of why we capture memories as we place value on the approval and praise of others who have nothing to do with the event. This in itself changes where our thoughts are during the event.

In the past, we cared deeply about how children felt as they saw their decorations for their birthday parties, or how a spouse would feel when he heard his big 40th birthday "Surprise!" Now, if it is not captured and shared, it didn't happen. We all have seen images of birthday parties and other events in which everybody at the event is holding a smartphone to take the perfect picture; their positioning and their observation of the event is all colored by taking the perfect image. The value of the event itself and the momentous occasion is somehow diluted. Instead of making being in the moment a priority, we make creating a moment to be *share-worthy* a big priority for the event.

Let's look at a scenario that will serve as a powerful illustrative analogy:

You plan a fall photography session. You have picked the perfect outfits for the whole family. A few minutes before the photographer arrives, your husband states he does not want to wear the outfit you chose. You are quite upset because you chose the colors deliberately and this is not the first time your husband had seen the color options. He refuses to even wear option two and now you are down on time. The discussion continues and gets elevated.

He thinks you planned this when he was not that interested. You think he does not appreciate the time you took to plan something for the family. You are controlling. He is inconsiderate.

The photographer arrives, your husband chooses what he wants and you continue with the photo session. Inside you are brimming with resentment; outside you are smiling because you paid for the photo session and you are not going to waste it— the perfect synchronization of great weather and well-behaved children not complaining about their stiff collars and sweater vests. The session is over. The day continues, and you do not have the energy to discuss the exchanges that took place earlier. You receive the pictures the next day. They look amazing. You post them.

Fabulous! In four hours, so many of your social media friends say wonderful things. The pictures are a hit! The husband's outfit was not really noticed as not matching the theme and you can relax.

Later that evening as you sit with a cup of coffee looking at the images one by one, you look closer at each picture. You remember that you yanked your child several times to get him in the right pose. When one child said she wanted to use the bathroom, you hushed her and told her to wait. You see that your husband put his arm around you but because you hated the color of his sweater, you decided to just take the picture; you didn't feel like leaning your head on his shoulder like the photographer suggested. And then all the things said come rushing back to you. What you said, and what he said. How you did not resolve it. You also feel you could have been a little nicer to the kids. After all, this was a family photo shoot. You could have laughed more, breathed more and hugged more. You feel guilt, and know there is some unfinished business to tend to.

Then the numbing starts. You remember the photoshoot was a success. You automatically start looking at the comments and realize that all is well. You are not going to discuss what was exchanged between you and your husband; you are just going to enjoy the fruits of your labor.

This is a good way to make it all balance out…until it happens again: another discussion where both you and your husband are on opposite sides, and you will bring up the photo session. And he will be surprised because he thought all was well because you were happy with the pictures.

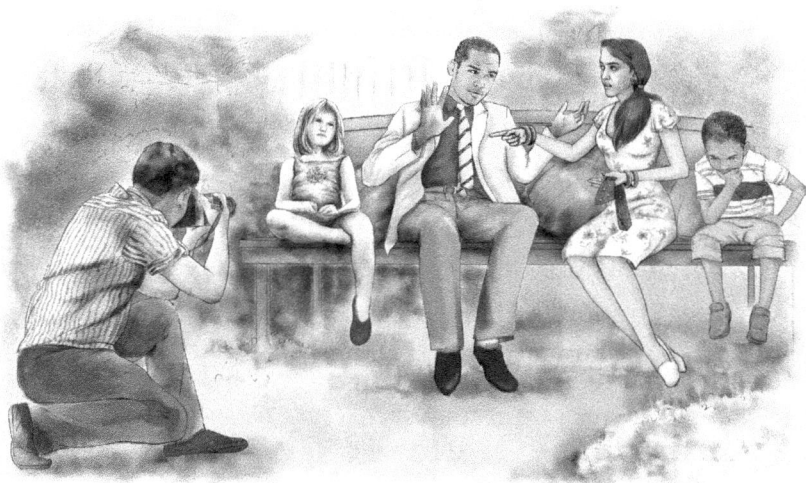

In this scenario, what if you made it a goal to make this session a memorable time for your kids? Instead of focusing on the pictures and obsessing that your friends already had great pictures last year, you just hug and kiss your kids and roll around with them in the grass? What if you actually did lean on your husband's shoulder, remembering that even though he did not follow the uniform code, he is alive and well and by your side?

What if, after the photo session, instead of putting so much effort into deciding which photos get posted online you had put some effort into having a discussion with your husband so you could both articulate your feelings? Maybe apologize to your little ones for being so dismissive?

Do you see the difference between the two approaches? Putting emphasis on the event itself, rather than the outcome, has everyone involved being present in the moment, even enjoying it. One approach takes you to growth and authenticity in your relationships while the other simply airbrushes your feeling and your misgivings.

Informational Overload

Social media and online news services have made everything more accessible and at your fingertips. The pro is that we do not have to wait very long to find out the latest update on the happenings around us and around the world. The con is that information is often fed to us in rapid form and the topics range from humorous to serious, very serious and downright tragic.

This causes us to scroll down our newsfeeds and see a wide variety of articles on the joys and losses in other people's lives. We are elated when we see a child with autism had the whole neighborhood attend his birthday party, allaying his mother's fears that nobody would show up. We are thrilled when an elderly gentleman survived transplant surgery after his daughter donated her kidney. We are sad when we see a transgendered teen bullied at school, but inspired when that teen takes on the bully through social media.

How did you feel reading these newsfeed topics? Do you see the range of emotions you felt in just a few seconds? Women are reading such a variety of news headlines (small, big, mundane) in the span of a few hours every day.

Studies show that when people are exposed to even the slightest image of a tragic event it stays with them for at least 24 hours. There are, of course, positives to this, as it develops empathy, a feeling of connectedness to community, and collective responsibility. The difficult thing for women today is finding the balance between the tragic and positivity. Women have told me that sometimes the tragic posts they see weigh so heavily on them that they cannot function, and then they immediately feel guilty when they click on something uplifting to escape the depressing feeling.

Here are a few tips on how to have a more balanced approach for your newsfeeds. When you see a shared news post's headline, decide whether this going to:

- Make me learn something I am actually interested in?
- Give me an update on something that personally affects me?
- Give me information on a topic that will make me smarter as a person about the world outside my immediate community?
- Give me an uplifting boost that will make my day go better?

If none of these four items check out, skip the news post. When you see a post or photos from a friend on your newsfeed, decide:

- Is this a close friend of mine who would have shown me these pictures in person? (Often people share with friends of friends without realizing it.)

- Do I enjoy this person's company? This will help you view the pictures from a positive place, because as you may understand already, whatever energy you put out by viewing something from a negative place usually comes come back to you.

- Will this brighten my day? Many people are going through personal struggles. Life has its seasons of ups and downs; if you are in an emotional season, protect your heart. For example, if you are trying to conceive and are having trouble, don't spend hours looking at someone's beautiful baby shower pictures. If you had a parent just pass away, try to temporarily avoid profiles that post a lot of parent-child pictures. It is ok; you will get there. Know your heart and what makes it sad or glad for the season you are in.

The bottom line is that you are blessed with 24 hours in a day. Make how you consume information count. If it does not uplift you or make you smarter or more globally aware, skip it.

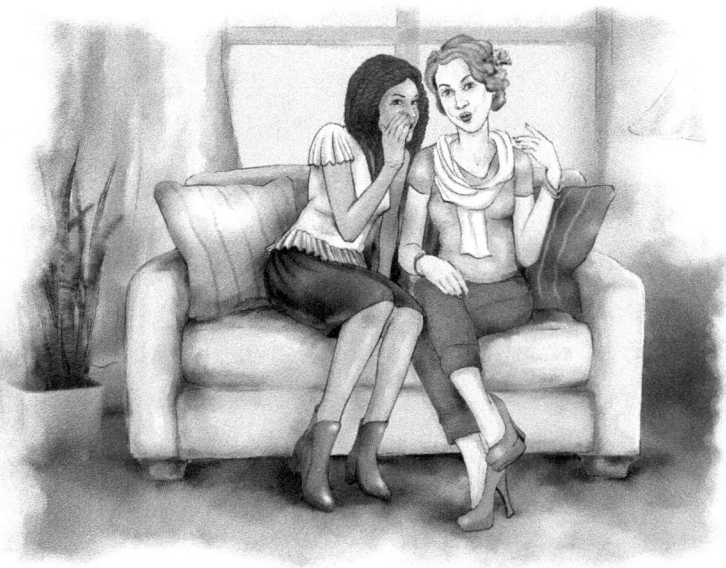

Chapter 5
TOXIC FRIENDS

According to the Urban Dictionary, a toxic friend is someone who "embarrasses you in social situations in order to gain attention; a person who betrays your trust; a type of friend who is OK one-on-one, but will turn on you as soon as other people are around, making it hard to break off the friendship...."[3] We can add behavior patterns such as inconsiderate, self-serving and competitive.

[3]Toxic Friend. (n.d.). Retrieved from http://www.urbandictionary.com/define.php?term=Toxic%20Friend

In her article, "Intimate Friend Circles Linked to Increased Happiness, Studies Show," Misty Harris reports that adult women have regular social media interactions with multiple Facebook friends, but only really have two or three close friends. Just like social media, any interaction online or in person needs to be monitored, and if it harms you, it's time for a detox.

Why We Keep Toxic Friends Around

Before we start the detox of unhealthy friendships, we must analyze:

- How they came to exist.
- Who they actually are.
- Why women gravitate toward them.
- Why women keep them around.

Messages in Childhood

I do not believe that women by nature are drawn to conflict. I do believe, however, that young girls develop an emotional awareness that allows them to experience stronger feelings than their male counterparts. Today, if you watch an episode of *Strawberry Shortcake* or *My Little Pony,* you will see plot themes of jealousy, competition, turf wars, and then, eventually, apologies. It seems that the most entertaining topics for young girls lately are centered on managing complicated relationships. I do believe these "harmless" cartoons are teaching young girls about these emotions and girl dynamics in a negative manner.

Many mothers have told me they have had to speak to their daughters about tools to deal with emotions in a positive way because the media is providing the constant opposite—true since the beginning of fairy tales. Why are all the negative characters in Cinderella female? The story deals with two jealous stepsisters, a conniving, ambitious stepmother, a helpless Cinderella and a prince who is above it all.

Since childhood, females have not been given proper guidance on how to handle the tricky emotions that come with a heightened emotional awareness and its interplay with interactions. This affects all personal relationships, but most definitely the ability to maintain strong and loyal friendships because, in the case of friendships, loyalty is not derived from bloodlines.

" My parents taught me at a young age that they were proud of me as long as I tried my best. They never stressed the end result; they always focused on the effort. "

Sarah Kureshi

How Toxic Personality Traits Come into Existence

Traditionally, the alpha female in any youth setting has not been the nurturer. She has been the competitor, the champion, and the popular personality. This is not by design, of course, but by nature. There has to be a leader of the pack among these young girls.

Childhood years and teenage years are marked by discovery of one's self, talents and ambitions. Thus, unless a child belongs to a particularly mature, introspective set of parents who have a lot of time to discuss emotional intelligence, most young girls are learning on the go.

The ultimate overachiever, Dr. Sarah Kureshi, holds a medical degree from Mayo Clinic, a masters in Public Health from Harvard University, and she was an NCAA All American Track Star and a Professor at Georgetown Medical School. Sarah Kureshi is a passionate medical physician who has traveled the world helping others. She is also a human rights advocate who rallies against violence against women.

Sarah has an interesting take on the importance of good parenting. She says, "My parents taught me at a young age that they were proud of me as long as I tried my best. They never stressed the end result; they always focused on the effort. I think because of that I never felt pressured and I was able to go along my journey without much stress. Also, there's something about 'not winning/not getting what you want' that really builds character and strength. So either way, it's actually a win-win situation. If you're passionate, motivated and dedicated, you can do anything you want to."

Not every girl reaps the benefits of positive parenting that focuses on personal development, integrity and character. The popular girls are usually too busy with social obligations, academic pursuits, and athletic challenges to have time to practice being nice. They are not deliberately being mean; they are deliberately busy trying to be the best. Those they deem as not "in their league" are going to feel the inorganic effects of their self-proclaimed superiority. Others girls begin to mimic the popular girls' behavior, creating a domino effect of toxic behavior. Girls at a young age see popular, competitive, self-serving personalities as winners.

It is not the popular girls who become toxic personalities as adults. Who are these toxic women, really, if not the mean, popular girls of the past? They are the girls who modeled the popular personality. Those girls—the ones who were on the sidelines—are the ones who later become adult toxic personalities. Think about it: are the toxic friends in your life the ones who have been at peace with who they are, or are they constantly struggling to figure out who they are, which yields to erratic, inconsistent behavior? When you speak to them, do you hear conversational styles that remind you of high school? There is a reason for that, as toxic friends are still mentally living in the past. Toxic friends are those individuals who have been social outliers, and they are hell-bent on not becoming those outcasts again. Let me elaborate more clearly. Have you ever heard the phrase, "If you are really something (whatever it is), you do not have to work so hard to prove it"?

By practicing what they perceive as the behavior patterns of popular people (winners), they allow toxic characteristics to develop and flourish in their adult lives. Most social circles have a toxic personality that has found a way to become a queen bee; at least for a short time. The queen bee usually gets dethroned very quickly.

Why Women Gravitate Toward Toxic Friends

We all remember the scene in *Mean Girls* when Lindsay Lohan's character states, "I didn't understand it; the more she (the alpha female and also toxic personality) treated us badly, the more we liked it." Lohan's character stages an undercover operation to take down the queen of popularity in her high school, Regina Jones. She notices that although

Regina Jones was practicing all the behaviors of a toxic personality, she still had many followers, sympathizers, and supporters.

Why Women Gravitate Toward Toxic People

Toxic personalities are those who are struggling to not repeat being outliers of any sort again. They use toxic behaviors as tools to keep relationships that serve them best. People who gravitate toward toxic people will fall into two categories:

1. **Those who are genuinely people pleasers.** They have a problem saying NO and an even bigger problem telling their toxic friends that they have a problem. Their gravitation toward toxic friends occurs because they never want to be in hot water with anyone. They will continue to tolerate toxic behavior and even applaud it. But eventually they will begin to mirror the toxic personality. By turning a blind eye to the toxic behavior of their friends, and by keeping them close without honest discussions, they turn out to be insincere themselves.

Being a people pleaser often causes individuals to be inauthentic and to support problematic behavior. It's like allowing a toddler to have tantrums because you are afraid the toddler will take out his or her anger on you. What does that make you? A bad parent. You do things to serve yourself rather than to benefit your toddler. Much in the same way, if you are enabling a toxic friend, you are not being a good friend. You are applauding bad behavior.

2. **Those who need the toxic friend.** These are people who rely on the bad behavior of the toxic friend. Through manipulation and gossip, toxic friends have a wealth of information. They can do a lot of the dirty work because that's their general reputation. In addition, toxic friends have mastered the art of climbing the social ladder. The people around them are sometimes able to follow their friends up a few rungs, too. Have you ever noticed that toxic people have a lot of benign and loyal supporters? One needs the other. The toxic person needs cheerleaders and the needy friends need an ally to do their dirty work and social climbing for them. It's just that simple.

How to Detox From a Toxic Friend

The WHY

In order to make a goal to detox from anything, you have to believe that your life will be more fulfilling and productive without it. Think about all the negative energy and time you spend on reacting to, thinking about, and managing toxic relationships. You will have to confront the reality that your toxic friends are adults and your keeping them around says more about you than them. It says that you do not value your own contributions and time as a friend. It says that your words, energy, and efforts are available for anyone who gives you recognition, regardless of how much respect they give you.

There are real gems in this world. There are people with generosity, compassion and loyalty as their core attributes. These are the types of people who are going to bring real value to your life. Our time is limited on this earth. We should make it a goal to spend our days surrounded by people who lift us up and support us. Otherwise, we may look up one day, years from now, to find that we've spent years allowing negative people to drag us down by consuming our time with their neediness. You have to complete an honest assessment of your friendships. Even if they did lift you up at one time, if their season of contribution is over it may be time to move on.

The HOW

There are several approaches you can take to separate yourself from a toxic friend, and the best approach is the one that empowers both you and your friend. You always want to make moves that have a positive effect on your surroundings. So even if you are sharing some tough love, do it with grace.

For tough conversations, one-on-one meetings are best. They can always start out with a long email, but many times our tones are not accurately reflected in writing. Invite them over for lunch or meet them for coffee. Tell them about your concerns, and how you have seen a pattern of betrayal or questionable behavior. When they respond, hear them out. Let them finish their thoughts. It is quite possible they may even get emotional, or worse, they may start to attack you. In all circumstances, move the conversation forward. Tell them that you are turning a over new leaf in your life. You are working on improving your time here on this earth to bring love and positivity around you. For now, this is not a positive relationship, and you want them to focus on doing the same for themselves. In this manner, you are lifting your friends up as you navigate through your toxic relationships. Reaffirm that we are all flawed human beings and the thing that matters the most is what we are doing to correct these flaws.

Once we start focusing on what we choose to bring into our lives, then we realize that other people are not the problem. As you change, you are opening the door for your toxic friends to start changing, as well. Then start distancing yourself through your time and attention. As you are entering into a cocoon (as discussed in Chapter 1) give them an opportunity to do the same.

The Real Housewives Encourage Toxic Relationships

It does not help that the most popular mainstream television shows revolve around plots that encourage disloyal, manipulative and dishonest relationships between women. In 2015 alone, Bravo shattered ratings records of show premieres by raking in 2.8 million viewers for its popular show *Watch What*

Happens Live, in which celebrity guests weigh in on the interactions of *Real Housewives* cast members. In addition, the premiere of *The Real Housewives of Atlanta* raked in 3.7 million total viewers. In the last six years, we have seen shows such as *Madame Secretary*, *Commander in Chief* and *The Chicago Code*, all with A-list actresses in leadership roles, plummet in the ratings or get canceled. What shows continue to do well as a proven business model instead? *The Bachelorette* and *The Real Housewives* series.

What is it about the *Housewives* concept that makes it so amazingly popular? The fights, the gossiping, the subtle digs, and the competition on looks, money, homes, cars, kids, husbands, and of course, handbags. It is a raw image of how women can behave in the company of other beautiful and successful women.

Sincere conversations between women take place only rarely in the show. One woman who opens up her heart as a confidante ultimately can use that same information as ammunition against another's deepest secrets and insecurities. In this case, is reality mirroring art or vice versa? What messages are we consuming and perpetuating in our real lives to our own detriment?

Let's be honest: no person is without flaws. No human being is free of failings of jealousy, insecurity, and misguided competition. We are all trying to navigate through the complex circumstances that life throws at us. However, is it really fair to have a television show that thrives on showcasing a person's weakest moments? All the women on these shows have the capability of being influential, positive mirrors for other women by the sheer power they have from being on a national television show. They are businesswomen, wives of wealthy men with access to resources and connections, and former TV personalities, yet the only attributes the show helps them share are their biggest weaknesses.

Who makes these shows successful? Is it smart marketing and repetitive reruns that are generating high ratings? Or, do consumers drive the success? Have we, as viewers choosing to watch these embarrassing moments of real live women, allowed the industry to reaffirm that a woman will always choose a cat fight, a gossipy rumor and backstabbing girlfriends over an uplifting show that portrays women as strong, powerful leaders? I challenge that we indeed have.

We have developed an appetite for voyeurism that has allowed Bravo to market to a niche of unhappy, bored and jealous women who love to sit in their living rooms and watch other women fall from grace. If that is what we choose to consume and accept as definitions of good friendships in art, how are we possibly going to be able to have good non-toxic friendships in real life? The reason shows featuring strong women in leadership roles do not last is simple: women do not want to see them. We do not tune in to see strong women playing complex roles that challenge their possibilities. Rather, we tune in to watch the simple caricatures of crumbling egos.

There is a parallel in what we consume and how we behave. The reason toxic friendships last so long is because we do not want to surround ourselves with powerful women who will push us to be more. We want to surround ourselves with women who maintain the drama and help us validate our need for gossip and unhealthy competition. Bravo is considered a giant in the industry of media for women. Reality TV perpetuates toxic relationships. If you cannot completely eliminate it, like toxic friendships, recognize what purpose it serves in your life and minimize it.

If you just finished this section and feel righteous because you have now identified your toxic friends and are thinking, *I can't wait till they read this*, stop! You are part of the problem. Understanding your own toxic nature is seeing that it is based on circumstances in your life that direct your behavior. You must realize this to end toxic cycles. If you start freezing out your friends and talking about them to others without giving them an opportunity to change, then you have become the very person you wanted to avoid.

Be careful. Practice your boundaries, but come from a place of compassion.

> *There is nothing wrong with a great haircut and a new pair shoes. But they dress up who you are underneath the skin; not the other way around.*
>
> Elizabeth Lesser

Make the Material Girl a Has-been

The things cluttering your closet and home are also cluttering your mind. There is nothing wrong with wanting nice things. Appreciating fine art, luxurious furniture, and beautifully crafted handbags is a nod

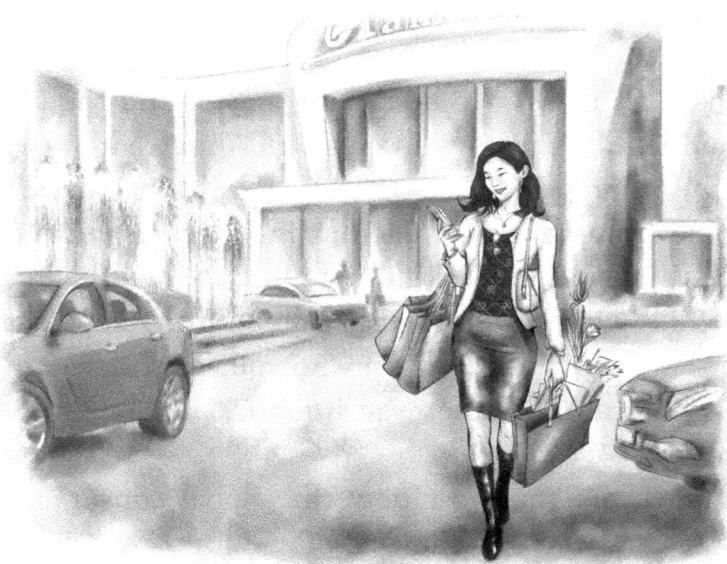

to the artists' vision. But this is not why a majority of women buy these items. Just look at the black market for designer goods. It is estimated to be a $500 billion industry. Thousands of retailers make a great profit by selling knock-off merchandise at low prices. This means, in essence, the seller of "Chanel" bags on a busy city street knows your purchasing tendencies more than you are willing to admit. They know you do not care about the artist's work. They know you want to be seen as someone who can afford luxury items. The majority of everyday, middle-class, working women and housewives are putting themselves in debt and consuming products more than ever before.

Elizabeth Lesser is a bestselling author and the co-founder of Omega Women's Leadership Center. She said, "Our power and influence and sense of self come from within—from our intelligence and our creativity and our feelings and our values. There is nothing wrong with a great haircut and a new pair of shoes. But they dress up who you are underneath the skin; not the other way around."

Women are the most powerful global consumers. What are we spending our money on? Here is an analogy. Imagine you were studying for a calculus exam. You would, no doubt, clear your Spanish flashcards and books from your desk to make room for your calculus materials. In the same way, you need to declutter your life to a make room for what's most important: you. Hence, we get the phenomenon of spring-cleaning or the nesting phase in which we start anew by getting rid of the unnecessary.

A new you needs a fresh slate to feel reenergized, focused and yes, detoxed. It is not an easy thing. The media and online advertising are constantly bombarding us, telling us we need more stuff. The reality is that we do not need more stuff. We need more us.

Regarding having more, publicist and author, Arielle Ford had this to say: "Having witnessed people in developing countries, people that we Westerners would consider 'poor,' these folks seem to have much richer lives. They have close family and community ties and are grateful for what they do have. They don't seem brainwashed into consumerism. And they live in a world where having 'enough' is all they need, unlike Westerners who always want 'more.'"

We cannot effectively start decluttering our lives of things unless we are honest about why we buy things in the first place. Women are buying for the following reasons:

1. They want people in their social circle to believe that they are powerful. This stems from their idea of what it means to be financially successful and what that should look like. The women who fall into this category grew up seeing others with

beautiful, expensive things and witnessed the buzz around these people. The buzz pointed to their being rich and powerful. These women want to feel like those women they envied.

2. They want to attract a certain type of person to their social circle. The women who fall into this category thrive on reflected glory. They feel if they surround themselves with rich people, everyone will understand that they, too, are rich and should be treated accordingly—with envy. These women pay for a handbag and shoes as advertisements of their connection with rich people.

3. They are under pressure to belong with the elite in their neighborhoods or social circles. These women want to be accepted. They may not even like the expensive handbags and clothes. But, they feel at the stage they are in their lives, they should be able to afford these items and belong in certain social circles. They use large purchases to validate success.

4. They apply a value to what it means to have expensive things. This category is the most problematic because these women believe the items define their happiness—define them.

Instead of focusing on interests, personality, development and sincere friendships, they believe people will like them for their things. And in turn, they will achieve happiness.

Our relationship with things is only harmful to us if it hinders us from being our true, authentic selves. Regardless of what category you belong to, all of the categories have one common unifying theme: they are a shield of protection to portray you in a certain way externally or fill a void internally. They are not just a manifestation of your appreciation for the goods themselves. Once we recognize the basis of our relationship with luxury goods, we can start the process of bringing this relationship into balance.

Gratitude

Consumption of things we do not need is directly tied to our contentment with what we already have. This contentment comes from gratitude. Gratitude is being appreciative of what we have and knowing we do not need anything more.

For many of us, gratitude is not a regular practice. We reserve the official time to be grateful when celebrating religious or cultural holidays such as

Thanksgiving. I have met many people who are swept into the wave of gratitude during such events. But then as soon as their daily routine takes over again, they are back to being pessimistic and stressed with life's demands. Hence, we get the phenomenon of "retail therapy."

If these words describe you, you are not alone. This state of being has become an epidemic and there is a good reason for it. Despite being one of the wealthiest nations on earth, with large pools of natural resources, we still have thousands of people living with anxiety, depression, stress, and debt.

Black Friday is just one example of how subtle messages through media and consumer-driven industries keep telling us that we need more things to satisfy an insatiable thirst. This is why as soon as Halloween is over, Thanksgiving sales start, and soon Christmas and Valentine's Day.

Everywhere we look our emotional attachment to special moments throughout the year is tied to purchasing power. So in reality, how can we really be grateful? The whole societal norm is to snap out of that gratitude nonsense as soon as possible so we can get right back to consumption and debt. The truth is, all the things we own are just things. They are expendable. All these items are lifeless. To quote Brad Pitt's character in *Fight Club*, "The things we own end up owning us."

People struck by natural disasters can be left helpless, and sometimes, homeless. What is it that makes them rebuild their lives, keeps them moving so they do not give up? "Things" don't actually save lives or help fill their needs. On the contrary, it is the bravery, sincerity, and care of the people around them that have helped them move along. It is the inner resolve that people develop and rely on to find joy again, not their fancy handbag, shoes, or big television that they went into debt for.

A few years ago, I had the privilege to attend a memorial event for my friend's sister. She was a young bride who was fighting cancer and very soon after she was married, she started to lose the battle and passed away. She was absolutely beautiful and always looked like a dignified fashionista every time I saw her. In addition, she was a very deep thinker and spiritual person.

At the memorial, my friend stated that her sister was known to be a shopaholic; she loved fashion and all its frills like most women do. As she was nearing her death, however, she changed her perspective.

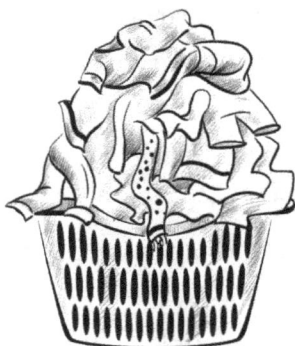

Realizing how fleeting life actually is, she started to see her things as a burden. She wanted to give away as many things as possible. In fact, she started giving away her clothing to her family members and would smile when she saw others wearing them.

The memorial itself was a charity auction of her most prized possessions of fashion and jewelry, some of which still had price tags on them. She also had my friend write down her thoughts as she was nearing the inevitable (as she could see the world differently than we could) and wanted to share her perspective with others after her passing. Below is one of the most powerful reflections shared with us (and there were many). I will try to quote the best way I can as to not insult her gracious intent to share:

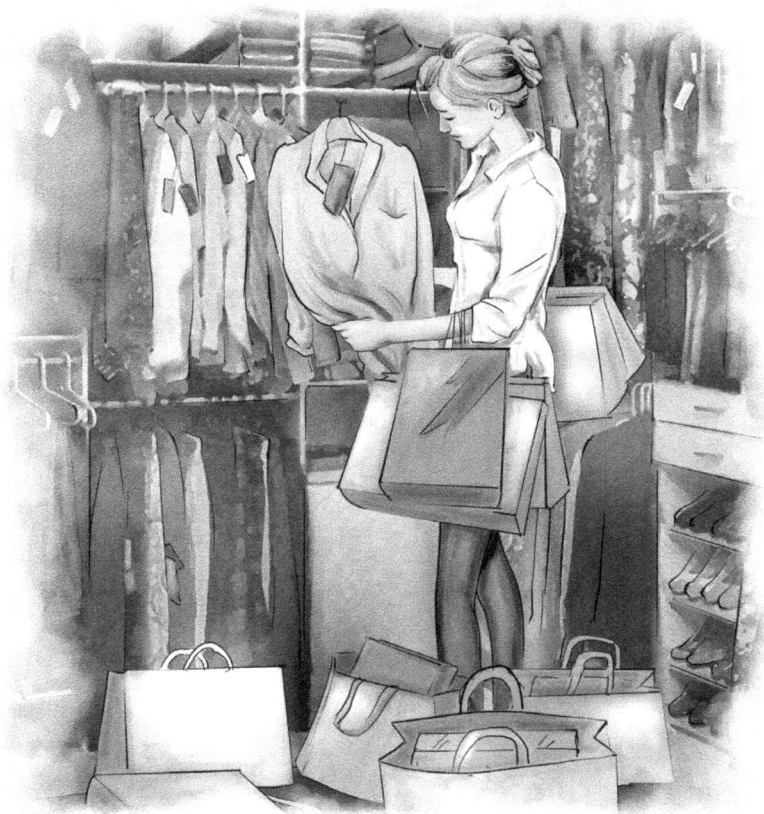

"Nothing goes with you after death. Only your relationship with people and the connection you hold with your creator. Things are just things. They are absolutely nothing. This is all nothing."

Powerful, indeed.

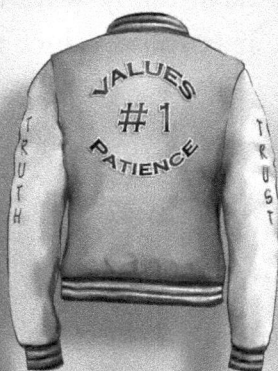

Chapter 6

WHO ARE YOU? IT'S A VALUES GAME

Here you are in your cocoon, in your reflective space. There are no friends to distract you, no media messages to define you. You are by yourself. Let's learn about you.

Is it a challenge to describe yourself, due to the presence of social media, targeted advertising, others' perceptions and stereotypes inundating our world?

Our goal should be the ability to describe ourselves with ease. We all have many sides to us, yet we all have core values. It is these values that define who we are.

> *" To me, healthy living is living in a way that leaves you feeling empowered, energized and enthusiastic about your life. "*
>
> *Pilar Gerasimo*

We delve into behaviors that are reactions to emotions we are feeling. But these behaviors and emotions are not our values; they are only reactions. Do you notice that as things have become more complicated and busy in our society, so have people? It follows, then, that when we are decluttering our lives through a deliberate detox of negative people and distracting things, we should also declutter our word bank. Keep it simple.

Values guide our words, actions and decisions. Living according to values is necessary for leading a healthy, fulfilling life. "To me, healthy living is living in a way that leaves you feeling empowered, energized and enthusiastic about your life. It's making daily choices that endow you with plenty of vitality, confidence and resilience to show up for the people and projects that matter to you. Basically, it's treating your body with respect, living in integrity with your priorities and values, and understanding the way your health is essential to them," says Pilar Gerasimo, the founding editor of *Experience Life* and *A Manifesto for Thriving in a Mixed-Up World*, a richly illustrated, award-winning chapbook about the guiding truths of the emerging healthy revolution.

Step 1: Peel Back the Labels

When my daughter was born, I was very deliberate about what messages she received about herself. I knew, as a female, that many people would be out to define her, to tell her what her place was, and what her interests should be. Even the toys available to her would be a certain color and would focus on activities such as brushing a doll's hair and ironing clothes. You would never see a child-sized ironing board in a boy's toy aisle. I remember when I was in the second grade, all the students were to choose instruments to play in the band. I chose what I thought would be the easiest to play and would come naturally to me: the drum. And who was trying out for the drum? Four boys and me. You can guess what I heard from the boys about my decision, but I was determined. And yes, to end the story on a good note, I was the one picked to play the drum. Never mind four weeks into band practice, my mother made me quit because lugging the big bass drum on and off the bus was just not good for my tiny second-grade body. This was just a one of hundreds of stories where other people would have an opinion on my choices of interests.

Armed with these memories in the 21st century, I wanted to give my daughter the tools to use her own vocabulary to define herself. So, I started early. When she was five, as I would put her to bed, I would ask, "What kind of girl are you?" She would repeat back to me, "Confident, brave, funny, and kind." In addition to stories of the little tugboat ("I think I can") and "Sticks and stones will break my bones but others' words will never hurt me," I have been getting positive messages across every day.

One day we were visiting a friend who remarked, "Oh, is she shy?" as my five-year-old daughter was hiding behind my leg. I replied loud enough that my daughter could hear me, "No, she is never shy. She is just picky about who she speaks to."

The more you tell a girl she is someone, the more she will believe you. We have to make a deliberate effort to take control of the labels we use to describe ourselves: make them positive and peel back the negative. There are many labels that people put on others that actually are positive, but are used negatively. Recognize the pure irrelevance of other people's labels for you so you are not motivated to internalize them.

> *Failure only exists as a perception. Everything is a lesson. What may seem as failure now, can seem as a blessing with hindsight.*
>
> *Ana Flores*

Let's look at a couple examples:

Power-driven
A thesaurus offers these synonyms for power-driven: exciting, electrifying, magnetic, and stimulating. These are all descriptions of people whom others would want to be around. But how is power-driven used about women in a conversational context? It means she only cares about herself. She wants control. She wants to tell others what to do. Is that not what we usually hear? It doesn't match with the textbook description, does it? That is because society puts baggage onto labels and then applies it to describe others to the extent where people actually start believing it. Let's talk about power-driven a little bit more because this book is written to specifically empower women. Why is having power or wanting power a negative? Whether it is launching a charity, starting a company or being the best mother you can be, you want to have the POWER to do that. You want access to do that. And that is not somebody who only wants to tell people what to do or to control people; it is someone who wants to control her destiny. When we use positive labels, these same people are called visionaries.

Failure:

When asked for a few words about failure, Ana Flores, who graced a 2010 cover of *Hispanic Business Magazine* as "The New Face of Social Media," offered this little gem: "Failure only exists as a perception. Everything is a lesson. What may seem as failure now, can seem as a blessing with hindsight. Confront the fear of failure head on and what results is a renewed sense of confidence."

Have you ever noticed that the 'F' we received in grade school when they still had paper quizzes and tests, was very similar to the 'A' in *The Scarlet Letter*? If you ever received an F, it would invoke feelings of shame, embarrassment, and low self-esteem. If someone else calls you a failure, it stings you even more. You feel you did not meet somebody else's standards. But here is the truth: no successful person has ever become successful without failing. Failure is where you learn more about the error of your ways or your mode of operation. It is an arrow to help you find your way to the correct destination or method, tweaking and improving on your skills. Failure, as a negative label, reminds you of your inadequacies. Failure as a positive label is your first necessary step toward success. See the difference?

> " *...I get so deeply engrossed in my projects, and am not able to take a step back to get perspective until I'm done with the work. When I complete a project, there is the fear that it isn't perfect...* "

Malika Ameen

Perhaps you did not have someone giving you positive labels to counter the negative ones as you were growing up, but it is never too late to begin. The first step in peeling back the negative labels is to identify them. What words make you feel uncomfortable that you have actually heard someone say about you? Which labels have you actually believed? Let go of them. Understand that nobody knows you more than you know yourself. A very practical exercise is looking at famous people in history. How many famous people were considered and labeled opposite of who they actually turned out to be?

Albert Einstein and Thomas Edison were both considered insane and academic underachievers by people around them; now they are celebrated as geniuses. How about Martin Luther King, Jr. and Malcolm X? Both were controversial figures in history and now are considered social justice champions. What about Susan B. Anthony? When she started championing women's rights in the late 1800s she was considered a nuisance and misguided advocate. The same goes for Harriet Tubman who courageously helped hundreds of slaves through the Underground Railroad. Today both of these women are considered pioneers. What people say about you has nothing to do with who you are. What they say is influenced by what their own reality and experiences are. You just have to be true to who you are, and getting to that is the most important part of the process.

Step 2: Distinguish Between Flaws and Negative Talk

Malika Ameen is a classically trained Chicago-based pastry chef and author of the recipe book, *Sweet Sugar Sultry Spice.* Like most women, she sometimes grapples with negative self-talk. I asked her recently about some of the fears she had in taking on a book project. She told me, "As a creative person, I get so deeply engrossed in my projects, and am not able to take a step back to get perspective until I'm done with the work. When I complete a project, there is the fear that it isn't perfect, that recipes and ideas need adjustments, or that an overall idea isn't as great as I think it is."

Ameen squashed those fears and silenced the negative self-talk. The result? Ameen's recipe book was a success paving the way for huge career exposure. She opened the critically acclaimed Aigre Doux Restaurant, where her dessert creations received high praise and accolades. Her restaurant drew attention from locals as well as influencers including Nate Berkus and First Lady Michelle Obama. She has appeared on national shows such as *Martha Stewart* and NBC's *Today Show*. Ameen also participated as a cheftestant in the inaugural season of Bravo's *Top Chef: Just Desserts*. She has been featured in various publications including *The New York Times* and *Food & Wine*. Ameen was able to soar because she recognized a perfectionist trait, but didn't allow negative self-talk surrounding it keep her down.

Our goal in our cocoon and path to transformative empowerment is to develop an honest conversation with ourselves about what we want to improve on. When I was in college, I used to make a list of different categories of how I wanted to improve my life. I would have one section that just focused on GPA, grades, and internship; another on health and fitness; still another regarding religious work (study and spirituality); and finally, personal attributes. The most comprehensive and significant category for me was grades and GPA, and getting the next internship.

The personal attributes were the easiest for me to write, but only because I was not very honest with myself. I kept describing my personality as some ideal and was never really admitting what I needed improvement on. What resulted was great success with some avoidable hiccups. The hiccups and low points came from the same mistakes I kept making again and again. Sometimes, I took opportunities I really did not believe in. Sometimes I advocated for issues that needed a different angle, and even though I knew the angle better than anyone, I failed to follow my gut instinct.

There have been times when I failed to take the advice of others. And, sometimes I have let negativity and others' insecurity-driven opinions of me go to my heart. These are scenarios that transcend the personal and professional realm, and they are not unique to me. I realized that if I am not working on improving my personal skills, then I would literally remain a hamster on a wheel in my relationships, my business dealings, and yes, my relationship I had with myself. This all stemmed from my having resistance to accepting my own flaws.

We should be OK with having a category in our life plan that says "flaws," those personality habits formed by years of doing things a certain way and reacting in a certain manner. I deliberately use the word "habits" and not "attributes," because habits can always be changed—and that is where we want to be headed, in the direction of changing our flaws to result in positive permanent attributes that become our core values.

I want to stress the significance of flaws because many will sugarcoat their reality. We fear that when we call out flaws in others or ourselves, we are perpetuating negative feelings. I disagree. Flaws are real; they are habits that need to be changed to better your life and you must take accountability for them.

For example, take toxic personalities: are we just being negative in our perspective if we call someone toxic? Of course not. Those who are constantly lying, manipulating and using people to serve their needs have serious flaws and have to confront their toxic tendencies. That is the only way we can transform in a productive way: to embrace flaws and forgive ourselves for having them. Once you recognize them, make a plan to change flawed habits. They say it takes three weeks to change a habit. Take the challenge. Every time you see that one of your flaws is creeping up, decide to take steps to eliminate it.

APPLY THIS TO YOURSELF

If your flaw is that you only care about things that relate to you, somehow (your egocentric tendencies), take steps to diminish your ego. When in a conversation with someone, ask him about his interests, ask for her opinions, inquire about others' daily activities rather than just focusing on your own. Commit to the whole conversation—to learning about the other person. Do this for 30 days in every conversation you have. What you will realize in the process is that you have missed out on a lot about the other person, and probably robbed yourself of an opportunity to learn something new. Just like any habit, you must make a deliberate attempt to break the chain of repetition by changing your behavior.

Negative talk is different from flaws. Negative narratives you replay in your head will sabotage your own success in your personal and professional life. Here are some examples that illustrate the differences between a flaw and negative talk.

Flaws:
- I am too quick to judge other people's intentions.
- I relate to everything as significant as long as it relates to me the same way.
- I get jealous of other people's success and start analyzing my minor accomplishments.
- I let stereotypes impact my friendships with people.

Negative Talk:
- I will never get that job. I am way too under-qualified. They will probably laugh me out of the interview.
- I will never be able to lose this weight. Nothing comes easy for me like it does for other people.

- I am just not good in relationships.
  I am probably better off alone.
- I don't know why I thought I would be a good mother. My kids will resent me when they grow up.

Do you see the difference? Flaws are personality habits. Negative talk relates to whether you will succeed or fail, focusing on how you will be perceived.

Of course, the biggest difference in the two is that the first one focuses on your present personality habit and the second focuses on your place in this world.

Negative talk is a destructive narrative that gets in the way of accomplishing whatever goal you set for yourself, big or small. Learn to remind yourself that negative talk doesn't equal facts. Negative talk is a false narrative that your insecurities create for you when you need an excuse to not push past your comfort zone.

Pushing past our comfort zones is what takes us to our destiny. We cannot afford to rely on a false narrative that holds us back. As Eleanor Roosevelt said, "You must do the thing you think you can't do." The simple way to not let negative talk enter your space is called the 3R Rule:

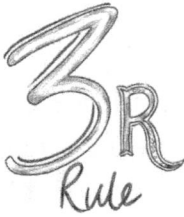

- Recognize you created it
- Reassess why you created it (are you running away from a challenge?)
- Run past it

Step 3: Decide What Your Values Are

Now that you: (1) have stripped off the labels that others have put on you; (2) identified what your flaws are and decided to fix them; (3) distinguished between your flaws and negative talk; and (4) recognized, reassessed, and replaced the negative talk; you are ready to decide what your values are.

What are values? Values are principles or standards of behavior—one's judgment of what is important in life. I like this definition because it puts you in the driver's seat in deciding what is important to you. This is the basis of you starting your transformation proactively.

In college, I would write my life plan, called positive goals. This was a list of things I wanted to be as an adult. It was not tied to my ambitions or professional goals, but rather to my spiritual path and "big picture."

You can do this at any point in your life. You can decide what core values you will stick to. (You can also consider them your principles.) The simpler the list is, the simpler your life will be, and the easier it will be to stick to these core values when you find yourself in unpleasant situations.

Now here is a simple question:
What is important to you?

Before I started my journey as an advocate for personal development, the world of serious spirituality and social entrepreneurship, I was headed in a completely different direction. Throughout junior high, high school, college and law school, I was Student Body President. Yes, I was that student. I was in love with school, student elections, campaigns, speeches, and ideas. In college, I had the ability to make an impact with my interests. I would advocate for diversity, minority recruitment, and allocation of funds to facilities for the disabled—even police brutality and wrongful arrest on campus.

For those who cannot appreciate student politics, student leaders founded every big civil rights movement. These student leaders spoke out on issues without fear of termination. The same followed when I became Student Body President in law school, where I advocated for teacher evaluations and diversity.

After graduation, I worked on creating political coalitions, wrote legislation for disadvantaged communities, and lobbied legislators. My work gave me access to legislators, political funders and real movers and shakers in politics. Everyone around me saw my trajectory toward having a thriving political career. Being a woman from a diverse background and being able to navigate complex legal/policy issues, along with personal relationships with political funders, made this path a very easy one to launch into.

Then I got a real taste of the political world, away from just the policy writing, advocating and making thoughtful arguments. I was hired to be a political director for a campaign of a person I admired. I fell into the work deeply, bringing resources, making introductions, and more. I was on a mission to contribute as much as I could.

However, eventually, I started seeing people I respected and admired taking steps I could not support. It was not that people were changing; the system was broken by design. I saw between the lines of what is ethical and what is legally permissible. After a very tough series of unfortunate scenarios, I exited from the environment. It was a crude wake-up call. After I was outside the situation, I concluded that the environment for me was too toxic. It was not good for my soul, nor did it agree with my values. I realized the world of politics at that time was not healthy for my personal spiritual path and ambition. I still wanted power to change the world and make a huge global impact, but I was going to do it on my ethical terms.

I went on to a start a company with a global mission that empowers women and gives me the platform to advance narratives I felt were missing from mainstream discourse. If you are reading this and my words and my example lift you up, then the impact has begun in a real demonstrative way. You would think that walking away from a professional world that I had been building up to since grade school would be the hardest thing to do, but it was quite the opposite. Once I identified my values and decided to make my life decisions based on them, it just felt like breathing.

I could not have discovered an alternative if I had not created a cocoon for myself. I embraced my flaws, my attachment to accomplishments and what I had thought was the only destiny for me. I came to realize that I could have a balance of many destinations. I deliberately replaced my negative words with positive ones. I owned what I considered important. My values are honesty, perseverance, optimism, and sincerity.

What are yours?

REFLECTION

- Peel Back the Labels

- Distinguish Between Flaws and Negative Talk

- Decide What Your Values Are

« Everyone has flaws and they are our beautiful imperfections that we can constantly improve on. They allow us to get in touch with ourselves and focus on personal development. We can be authentic by being transparent when necessary. »

Maaria Mozaffar

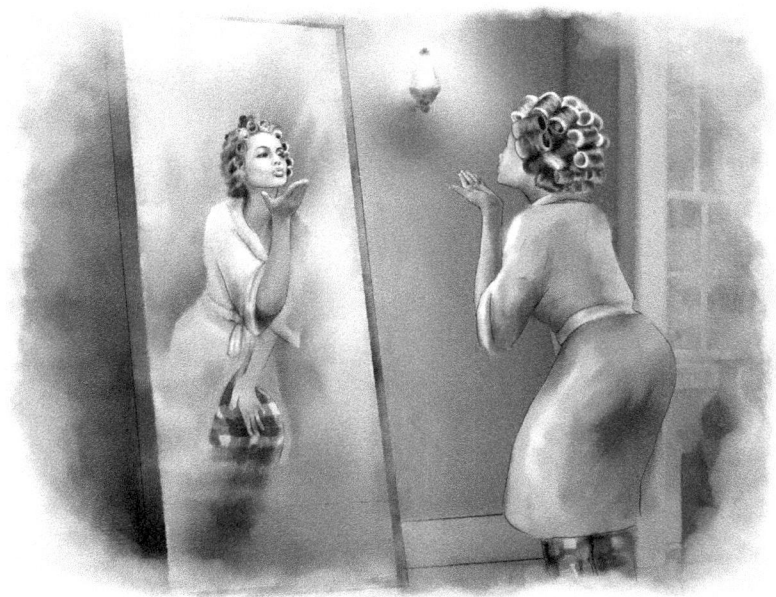

Chapter 7

PERSONAL POWER

"Power" carries a negative connotation when associated with women. Women having power should be something we as a society encourage.

Powerful people are generally thought to be loud, bold and center stage; however, personal power does not have to look like that. Personal power comes from (just as the name states) your own space.

We weren't taught to acknowledge ourselves. Very often, girls were taught that speaking well of themselves was bragging. There's a distinction between acknowledging ourselves and bragging.

Marci Shimoff

I define personal power as the control you have over your actions and the thoughts that serve you. It is the power you have to make your decisions. When asked for an opinion, you have the authority to be unapologetically honest about where you stand, and when challenged to act you have the power to act. Personal power plays a role in the moments when you have a conversation one-on-one. You remain clear and truthful to your perspective—and absent sound logic and wisdom, you cannot be persuaded for the sake of peer pressure.

Marci Shimoff is a NY Times bestselling author, a celebrated transformational leader, and a leading expert on happiness, success, and unconditional love. When asked why women don't take time to appreciate their own power, she said, "We weren't taught to acknowledge ourselves. Very often, girls were taught that speaking well of themselves was bragging. There's a distinction between acknowledging ourselves and bragging. Bragging is saying, 'I'm the best, nobody's better.' But acknowledging our self for qualities that we appreciate about ourselves is a very vulnerable act. To say I appreciate myself because I'm a loving person, or because I'm competent at my job, is not bragging. It's merely telling the truth about our own strengths."

Why is personal power so important? Well, without it you cannot be who you are. If you do not have the power to be yourself, you might as well imitate a stranger. There are three areas that one needs to work on to begin the process of harnessing one's power:

- Setting Boundaries

- Developing Self-love

- Striving for Authenticity

Setting Your Boundaries

Throughout time, societal expectations have made it all too easy for women to give away their personal power, and thus not protect their boundaries. Without boundaries, people do not accurately understand emotional, physical, mental and moral limits. Anyone who has a relationship with you should understand his or her boundaries.

Take a simple example: the pressure to be accepted as a nice girl. Let's first flesh out the word "nice" itself. Nice is defined as pleasant, agreeable and satisfactory. The word is an adjective. Technically, if one is nice, one is always pleasing, agreeing with, and satisfying others.

Is that really what women should strive to be? If we were to follow this description, we would never have any meaningful conversations or honest exchanges of ideas. In a nutshell, if practiced, this definition would halt us from growing.

People-pleasing
According to this definition, nice becomes an instrument to enable you to be satisfactory to others. What is this a symptom of? Yes, the dreadful

disease that takes over every woman starting as early as childhood: people pleasing. We know all too well what happens when women fall under the pressures of this act. Women by nature want to always keep the peace, which is admirable. However, the habit of being nice at the cost of your own emotional health can be dangerous. It starts out with your need to be nice in your personal relationships to, in turn, be nice in every scenario, making it hard to set boundaries.

To give you an example of how this habit can reach beyond your emotional health, I want to share something that alarms me. I heard a radio interview with a police chief speaking about sexual assault. Do you know the number one reason why women are in danger? They invite the intruder in either by physical entry or by conversation, because they are afraid they will not come across as nice. I know this is a more dramatic scenario, but this goes hand-in-hand with women not being able to set boundaries.

Polite is Different from Being Nice

I believe you can keep the peace and maintain respect for others without becoming insincere. But to have your personal power, you must maintain your boundaries proudly.

As I have come into the adult woman phase of life, I have a greater appreciation for manners and rules of etiquette. Words and phrases that I found unnecessary and bothersome from my mother, I now have come to have great respect for.

You see, being polite actually gives you the tools to set your boundaries with grace. It is entirely different from being nice. It allows you to speak your mind with very precise, accurate words without speaking in half-truths.

Let me give you examples of statements made by a *nice* person:

- "No, I really didn't mean that. I am so sorry."

- "Oh, I don't care about that; don't be silly."
- "Sure, no, you are fine."

- "Really? I don't remember saying that. Don't worry about it."

Now, here are polite statements:

- "Thank you, but I am full."

- "No, thank you; it's not something I am interested in."

- "Let me finish what I am saying, please."

Do you see the difference? The practice of being nice is about satisfying the other person, while being polite is about speaking your mind.

Everybody's Friend Is Nobody's Friend

My mother used to say this to me, and I never understood it until I became an adult. Someone who is always trying to be nice to everyone will always be in a position of being in an insincere conversation. It is impossible to be nice to everyone at an equal degree because people, agendas, and loyalties differ. I would say that many people fall into this category, not realizing that it can harm their credibility. They put themselves in compromising situations and conversations that may be considered backbiting. We all intend to be equally friendly with everyone, but the best situation is to strive to be polite and thus have varying levels of friendship.

This gives you the freedom to step away from conversations that you do not want to participate in and still maintain a relationship that is sincere while giving others the opportunity to be the best of themselves. If you do not arm yourself with these boundaries, you will step into a less graceful version of yourself. And yes, we have all been there.

Teach children that being described as fair, polite and trustworthy puts them in a category of being useful to others. People will approach them for help if they have integrity. All relationships should be based on respect and honesty, not on a superficial exchange of two people not wanting to offend each other.

Developing Self-love

You cannot truly be powerful if you do not love yourself. I know this seems like an outdated topic, but the truth is, every day and everywhere women feel they are not good enough. This is why consumer-driven industries and powerful media and advertising are so powerful: they capitalize on our insecurities and bad days.

Gratitude

Close to my 30th birthday, I opened a magazine to find an advertisement for a face cream with the line, "Look like you are 29 forever." This experience said it in a nutshell. When we reach a great milestone in our lives, outside forces tell us what is not so good about us anymore. It is a really warped way of living, being, and receiving information.

To love yourself you need to get to the basics of who you are so you can appreciate your own history. I read the following quote yesterday:

"How cool is it that the same God that created the mountains, oceans, and galaxies, looked at you and the thought the world needs you, too?"

You have to believe in your heart that you belong in this world and your unique qualities have a purpose. The key to understanding the value of your worth is gratitude. Gratitude practiced daily and deliberately will protect you. Only then will you be able to overcome the constant external forces trying to convince you that you are not good enough.

Self-love Means Countering Negativity

Circumstances, past voices, and media messages defining a standard of beauty can impact your acceptance of yourself in a powerful way. Here are some real practical ways you can counter those negative sources that impede on your self-love.

Challenging Circumstances

Things don't always go your way. It could be as major as your home being foreclosed to as minor as your forgetting to pack your child's lunch for school. For women, both of these examples can weigh heavy on the heart and can lead to negative thoughts that make us feel completely inadequate.

Knowledge is power. Look throughout history for the people who have made a positive impact on this world. Many of them had crumbling marriages, failed businesses and other personal losses. Did this impact their contributions? Did they give up and go home? Just imagine if people you admire actually started believing that negative circumstances were there only to tell them they were not good enough. Consider Princess Diana: people loved her because she was a royal with a humanitarian heart. She challenged the way the Royal Family interacted with the mass population and tried to consistently break barriers between people and ethnicities.

However, she had a dark side. Despite having the best of circumstances financially, she also had a husband who visibly was not in love with her. She had thousands of paparazzi following her every day, wanting to make money off her every move. Think about that for just a minute.

The media's fascination with her life and marital problems were not her fault. Despite the public and embarrassing side of her personal life, she still went into crowds, hospitals, and orphanages, embracing her role, knowing what she needed to do. Her position gave her the access to do what she wanted to accomplish. Now, apply this to yourself.

Negative Past Voices

We tend to internalize the negative things people say about us to our own detriment. We lean into every voice that has ever told us that we could not accomplish something or that we are inadequate. They creep into our minds when we need them the least.

Have you ever heard of the phenomenon of selective hearing? I know every mother has. We need to apply the same practice to our past negative voices. To do that, you have to deconstruct the negative voice itself.

When I was in law school, I was having a lot of trouble with legal writing my first year. I came from a background of composing short fiction and political science pieces, and to write with brevity and analysis seemed so restrictive. My legal writing teacher asked me at the end of the year, "Well, you passed. You didn't achieve any high marks for this. Let me ask you, do you really want to be here?"

Bless her heart, she did not mean to be cruel, but those were not the words I wanted to hear when I just finished my first year of law school. I wanted to feel achievement and that I was prepared to go on to my next year. I answered in the positive and moved on to the next year.

Just a few months earlier I took a law school exam in which I had the same issue. I struggled to respond to a restrictive bullet point list on how to analyze a legal issue. My Torts professor at the time took me aside and said, "I had to give you this grade, but look, you need to analyze it a different way. It is clear that you understand the material well, but it is just not coming across on paper." I understood what he was saying. I heard "You are smart, you belong here, and you just need to tweak your writing so people can understand you."

When my legal writing professor served me some tough words, I went back to the words of my Torts professor and replaced what I was hearing. This is selective hearing. I did not totally discount what the negative voice was; I just deconstructed it, countering with the more positive information I received from my professor who also evaluated my skills. Armed with a past positive voice, I improved.

You can deconstruct a person who has said something negative to you, as well, rendering it almost worthless. By asking, Why did he say it? What frame of mind was she in? Isn't he judging without first walking in my shoes? Am I the same person now that I was then? and my favorite question, Has she never failed at anything? Unlikely. Once you ask the questions, you can try to understand where others are coming from and try to balance the bias and negativity. You can do this in your professional life and your personal life and then embrace your challenges from a place of power.

Negative Body Image

Both social media and mainstream media messages can be very damaging to our self-esteem and self-worth. Repeatedly we are seeing media messages defining what the standard of beauty is, and for ages beauty has been central to a woman's identity. One of my friends, who is a very successful fitness trainer, confessed to me, "When I look at ads, I feel so insecure. I feel great when I am walking around, but then I open up a magazine…"

There is such an emphasis on what we look like and what we should look like, that it affects how much we appreciate ourselves if we don't look like the ideal. I was watching a very successful female American politician on television. This woman is one who has broken glass ceilings in all her ambitions. As a guest on a talk show, she responded to the question, "If you were not who you are now, what do you wish you could be?" She responded, "Well, I will say I wish I could be America's Next Top Model…" Then she continued the interview, but what she stated in the first words of her response spoke volumes. Despite having so much power and success, she still struggled with the standard of her physical beauty.

We get pressured to be beautiful in a certain, prescribed way from childhood. My mother kept my hair short. As a toddler, this meant wild red curls. There are very few pictures from my early years where I am sitting like a pretty, proper girl with decorative clips in my hair. In fact, I remember always getting scrapes and new bruises on my knees.

As I grew a little older, my classmates had perfect pigtails or long ponytails. I remember looking at their flowing locks of hair, wishing I had the same. Instead, I had a boy cut, famously known as the "Diana Cut." Surprisingly (insert sarcasm), I looked nothing like Princess Diana. Instead, I looked like a skinny boy with bruised knees, with short black hair, wearing a dress. According to my mom, it was so I could enjoy being a kid—so I could run, jump, and swing from the monkey bars without having to worry about a ponytail or braids coming undone.

Finally, I started looking like a girl, but I still was not able to do what other teenage girls did. I was not allowed to wear lip gloss, blush or mascara all the way through high school.

Despite all the other girls giving into the definitions of beauty, I never felt ugly, and never even knew I was a Plain Jane. I never felt I needed concealer to conceal anything. Other than wanting long locks of hair, I was simply perfect in my mind.

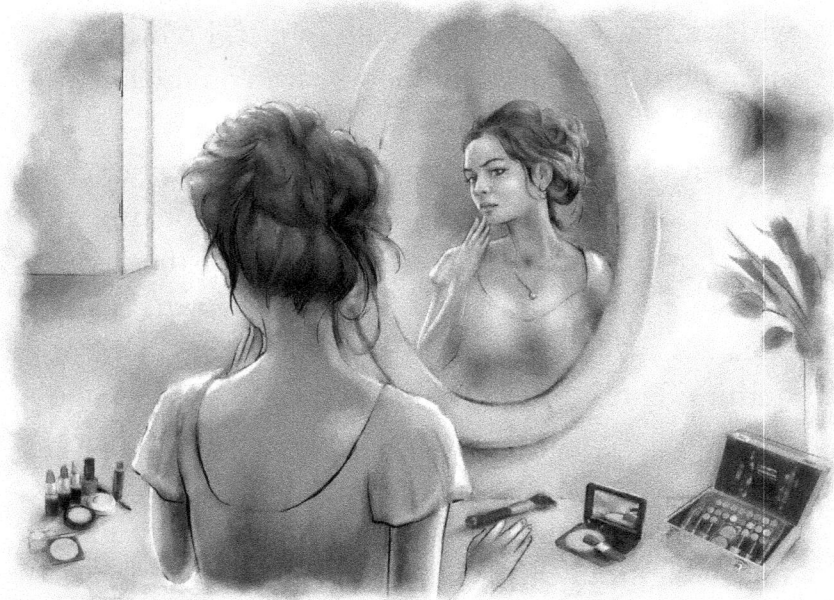

I was able to try so many new things, take risks and excel in so many different things in school that I must have honestly thought I was pretty amazing all the way around. I am not saying this to brag, I am simply analyzing how a Plain Jane, surrounded by beauty queens, managed to be a well-rounded, extremely confident young girl. I did not see myself the way I see myself in those photos now because I know the power of concealer, blush and eyeliner. I also did not see myself perhaps how others saw me.

I saw me how my mother saw me. My mother never called me beautiful. In fact, she never called anyone beautiful. My mother only talked about other girls as smart, funny, classy or confident. Thus, naturally I started to appreciate those qualities in other girls and wanted to emulate myself to be a girl with such attributes. In turn, others responded to me in kind. I thought I had it all and knowing that I knew they believed it too. What a lesson for life.

Beautiful was powerless to me. It was a word that had no value in my mother's eyes. It was a happy accident and perhaps why it was never impressed upon me.

When I look at my pictures as a teenager, I see the brilliance of it all. The calculated strategy my mother imposed on me to help me gain inner confidence without relying on my exterior. It was not until I reached adulthood, my mid-twenties, did I realize how others viewed me physically. It was through the eyes of strangers that I realized how much people respond and judge you on your looks. It was actually a disheartening reality.

Women are unnecessarily tough on others. Perhaps it is because a lot of women are victims of the cycles themselves; always feeling that they are not pretty enough. It is never too early or too late to break this cycle.

We should be beings of infinite power who are constantly building our inner strength and character and teaching the coming generation of the great value in these attributes. Looks fade; your power should be consistently growing stronger.

Striving for Authenticity

Authenticity is an unfiltered version of you. It is the ability to be who you are without the influence of others' expectations of you. In a nutshell, authenticity is your ability to behave according to your values. If you can align your actions and words consistently, you will find it much easier to use your personal power. If you are powerful, you will be able to be consistently authentic. It seems simple enough, but creating boundaries is easier said than done. We assume it will be an extreme overhaul of who we are and become intimidated when trying to gain authenticity. This book gives you a whole process to do just that: transform your life to be authentic. We can take little steps to help us stay authentic on a daily basis. Like all habits, authenticity must be practiced daily.

Speech

How many times have you been in a conversation and misstated your opinion just to go along with another person? Maybe you didn't intend to be fraudulent; it could be because you did not want to disrupt the flow of the conversation. I have witnessed this, especially if people experience a little social anxiety. I would suggest this happens when we are not pacing the conversation. Our speech travels with the same energy that the conversation demands and we think less about our responses. Of course, more serious incidents happen when we say things to people-please or to impress someone; these little white lies slowly lead to inconsistency in our own personal character. Remember, words are power: make them matter. Here are some simple tips:

- You can pace the conversation to your liking. Just because the conversation is going fast, it does not mean you cannot slow it down. You can ask people to "please repeat." This gives you time to gather your thoughts and actually hear what the other person is saying.

- Remind yourself that not all conversations need your input. You can be part of a conversation without speaking. You can nod and listen.

- Ask questions more than make statements. Have you ever heard the saying, "The smarter person listens"? The more you let other people speak, the more opportunity you have to consider and time your words.

Hearing

If you are present in a conversation that dishonors others, you are just as guilty of dishonoring them unless you put a stop to it. Much like speaking, you can, as a daily practice, hear what you want to hear and you will never feel that you were a bystander to bad behavior. This could be a benign conversation that misstates what type of job your friend has or something more serious such as a statement on someone's marriage or an attempt assassinate another's character.

Here are two simple tips for hearing no evil:

- Walk away.

- Tell the gossiping person to stop.

Being authentic as a person is a goal that includes little steps you do daily. Like building blocks of strength, do not underestimate their power.

REFLECTION

- Set Boundaries
  - People-pleasing
  - Polite is Different from Being Nice
  - Everybody's Friend is Nobody's Friend

- Develop Self-love
  - Gratitude
  - Self-love means Countering Negativity
  - Challenging Circumstances
  - Negative Past Voices
  - Negative Body Image

- Striving for Authenticity
  - In Our Speech
  - In Our Hearing

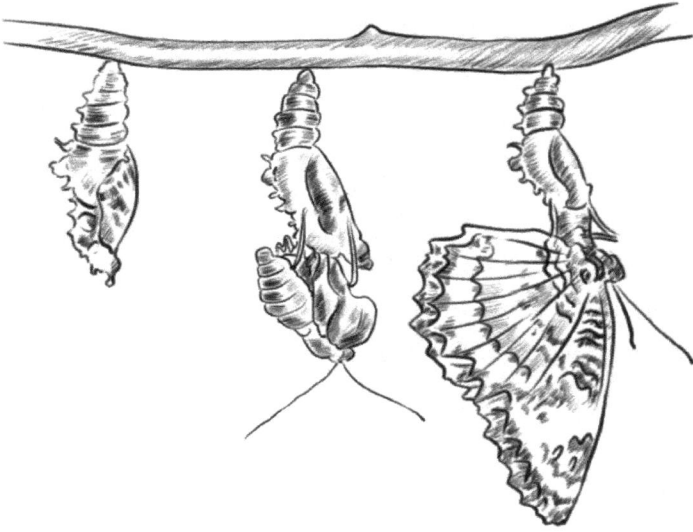

Chapter 8
TOOLS FOR TRANSFORMATION

Being powerful means being able to embrace your purpose. It means being able to show up to any challenge that destiny throws your way. However, if you are not in proper form to discover your purpose, you will never be able to fulfill it or even have the capacity to search for it. If you have chosen to take this journey, you have decided that you want to accomplish something big, to perfect your skills or take steps to become an extraordinary version of yourself. No matter what your finish line is, you have already set some goals for yourself. Goals are what lead you to your purpose, and to achieve goals you need creative, repetitive and skill-enhancing tools to take your ordinary days into the extraordinary. The more extraordinary your days are, the closer you are to building an extraordinary life.

Thus far, we have talked about mental shifts and altering how you think and relate to yourself and others. In this chapter, we will focus on physical and mental tools to help bring you closer to your goals. We are going to use a very simple acronym. Goals are as vital for a successful life as water and air are vital for you to live. Thus, we will call these tools W.A.T.E.R.—a lifeline to your extraordinary.

WAKE UP

Morning is defined as the first or early period of anything; beginning. Every morning we experience is a new beginning. Tomorrow, pause before you even open your eyes. Your day begins here—right here, as you open your eyelids. The way you approach this one action will set the tone for your day. When you wake up and open your eyes to the world, answer these important questions:

1. What and who are you waking up for?
2. What are you waking up from?

Joy and pain both have their limited time. Every time you awaken, you are leaving something that has a limited life. Figure out what you did the day before. How can you improve on that experience? Whose world can you brighten today?

Having a productive day actually comes from our ability to be grateful for little things. Every time you open your eyes, think about others who are not able to open their eyes. Just think for a moment about all those people who have slept their last night and seen their last day.

When I wake up every morning, I start my day by saying "Thank you." I look outside. I pause and admire the clouds, the colors of the sky, and the sun if it happens to be a sunny day. I reflect on how magnificent the sky and all its moving parts are, and how it sits above all the millions of people below, walking, thinking, planning and worrying. It reminds me of how small my "big" problems are in the big picture of our world. I also think there must be a reason I am still here. In this one moment, I think about how I am about to begin a new day to accomplish what I wanted to yesterday, to add new steps to my final goal, whether personal, spiritual or professional. I also pray—for guidance, for the ability to be grateful, and to maintain a connection with my Creator.

I heard the best quote in a coffee shop one day. One gentleman asked his friend, "It's Monday: are you ready for today?" The other man responded, "Yes. The question is, is it ready for me?" Wake up and plan to make the most of everything each coming day has to offer.

The outcome of a situation is not based on the circumstances that surround it, but rather on the attitude you bring to the circumstances. This is analogous to one of my favorite quotes from Tony Robbins: "The success of a business is not based on the amount of resources you have, but rather how resourceful you are." Being resourceful and having a good attitude allows you to be optimistic and creative with the intangible.

ATTITUDE

Some people always see the glass half-full. They are always looking forward beyond their obstacles and focusing on what they can improve, change and solve. We call these people the incurable optimists; we consider them, to the core, happy and positive. If you speak to optimists, they will tell you it is not just a personality attribute, but it is a daily repeated practice. They decide to bring an attitude of optimism to their day, to their obstacles and their circumstances.

I attended an inspirational talk given by a retired female Army general. She said even now when she enters a boardroom to speak, she gets nervous, but she decided to focus on positives. "No matter who I meet, I like them." How powerful! She found a way to make negative people, comments, and interactions completely irrelevant to her by maintaining a positive attitude toward them. It's not naiveté that keeps her from seeing negative traits in others, it's a choice.

Nobody exemplified this to me more than my mother. I never heard her say anything negative about anyone. When my siblings or I would comment that people she was socializing with had certain character flaws, she would simply make no comment and stay silent.

She did not want to engage and did not want to focus on the negatives. Similarly, deciding only to take the positives from every situation allows you the energy and freedom to continue with relationships, projects, and goals with a vision of success and completion.

One day, I worked very hard on developing a policy plan and finishing writing an important document for my company. Early in the morning, after dropping my daughter off at school, I stopped by the grocery store on my way to the productive day I was about to embark on. I thought, "How wonderful, that I could be this superwoman, multi-tasking mother."

After I loaded my groceries into my car, I turned the key in the ignition…and nothing. My car would not start. My battery died. I called roadside service and waited for them to jump-start my car. Then I located a nearby auto repair shop, drove there and bought a new battery, only to find out that, by mistake, they installed the wrong type, which caused a fuse to malfunction in the car, delaying my return home by about three hours. I did not have a charged phone any longer, and there was no Wi-Fi in the auto shop. This is a perfect example of how each day is indeed an adventure, and the only thing you are being tested on is what attitude you bring to the circumstances. In the early chapters of this book, I discussed SL (the

Second Level, where cognitive functions reside). The SL kicks in during challenging times. I sat there knowing there was some reason I was put in that predicament, and if I just used my FL (First Level, or physical response) to react to the situation, I would only end up frustrated and annoyed at the delay.

My immediate needs were to be quickly relieved of this situation so I could check my email, call someone or just go home. But I had decided earlier in the morning that I was going to be grateful and have an impact of some sort around me. So I did.

I maintained a positive attitude and used the time to take a breather, reassess my plans, and just simply marvel at the skill of the mechanic. I was surprised by how courteous, professional, and dedicated the mechanic was. I realized that every day he probably deals with many clients who are frustrated with their situations and yet, throughout our three-hour interaction, he was patient and yes, helped me stay relaxed by exuding an attitude of positivity. That is the lesson I was supposed to learn through the process: to see optimism and patience through the actions of another. If I had not chosen to have a positive attitude throughout that frustrating morning, I would have missed that learning opportunity. I would have also allowed the stress to carry through the rest of the day, which would have made it difficult to continue to get back to my tasks to accomplish my goals for the day, which consequently turned into the goals of the week.

The truth is, whatever circumstance or person crosses your path is a deliberate plan of the universe. It is up to you to decide to make your interaction with this situation or person an asset or liability for you, and then you take it forward from there.

Time

Twenty-four hours is a long time. It's 1,440 minutes, to be exact.

Do you ever notice that there are people, no matter what stage of life they are in, who are always out of time? They never have time for anything. They are perpetually stressed, perpetually tired and perpetually late. I have seen this in different scenarios and even in my life until I cracked the code.

Time is your most important asset. Every day you should be busy fulfilling your purpose, and to even discover your purpose, you must simplify your life.

Tips to Make the Most of Time:

1. *Let go of things that do not fulfill you.*
To have a life of substance, you need to get rid of distractions that are substance-less. How many ladies' lunches can you attend, how many shopping trips can you take, how many socialite events do you need to be seen at, and how many television shows can you watch that do not make you smarter? These are things that only serve as a distraction for us, and yes, they waste time. Whether your goal is to be the best caregiver, best advocate, best woman, best mother, best wife, or best professional, you need to dedicate yourself to developing skills. And for that, you need time.

Make an honest list. Cancel things that do not serve you and open up your days to discover what you are good at and how to become excellent at what you are already interested in. Do your days, weeks and months run into one foggy memory? That is a good sign that you are allowing precious moments to escape from you. Don't take this lightly. When you come across an activity that is draining you mentally and physically, with no sign of elevation in your spirit or skill, it's time to kill it. Replace that activity with a skill-building activity. Your interests will lead to your passions, and in turn, direct you to your purpose.

> " *Find your passion, find a way to monetize your passion and serve others. The compound effect of your daily activities will lead to success.* "
>
> Jacqueline Camacho-Ruiz

Jacqueline Camacho-Ruiz is an award-winning entrepreneur, media maven, national speaker, philanthropist and author of six books. She is founder of The Fig Factor Foundation, focused on unleashing the amazing in young Latinas. Jacqueline said, "Find your passion, find a way to monetize your passion and serve others. The compound effect of your daily activities will lead to success." When asked how to discover your passion, Jackie had this advice: "I discovered my passion by listening to my heart and paying attention to what made me happy. I was curious and relentless in finding my passion (asked questions, wrote in my journal, recorded my experiences, meditated to discover what fulfilled me) and today I live it every day."

2. *Slow down and be present.*
I learned the most about being present after I had my kids. I realized the moments that were simple routine chores for me were memories for them. I thought back to when I was growing up...when my mother set the table for breakfast...when she cuddled with me and spoke about the theme for my next birthday party, or how she smelled after she put on her nightly face cream.

This made me realize that little moments that may be inconsequential to me may be a memory for someone else or even a last interaction I have with someone else. A few years ago I lost an aunt to an illness. She was a vibrant soul who had traveled the world.

A week before she died, she left me a voicemail asking me how my kids were. I had many to do lists and never-ending chores, and she passed away before I could return the call. If I had only slowed down and taken the time to call her right away, I would have had the chance to speak to her one last time.

When you slow down and savor every moment, you will not only spend your time more efficiently but you will also become more productive, with greater focus and purpose. There is a myth that an efficient person is one who can multitask. However, the studies regarding brain activity[4], productivity and multitasking show the opposite.

MIT neuroscientist Earl Miller notes that our brains are "not wired to multitask well...when people think they're multitasking, they're just switching from one task to another very rapidly. And every time they do, there's a cognitive cost." When you attempt to multitask you are less productive and effective. Our brains are meant to do one task at a time and to be present.

When I finally made the shift to slow down in conversation, interactions, and work to be more present, I started holding on to many more memories. Nothing was foggy anymore. In fact, one of my cousins showed me a picture of my daughter from a while ago. When I saw the image, I knew exactly where we were the day the picture was taken. It is in these moments you realize that you are present and appreciate that each moment is an opportunity for a lasting memory.

---

[4]Heid, M. (2015, May 03). You Asked: Are My Devices Messing With My Brain? Time. Retrieved from http://time.com/3855911/phone-addiction-digital-distraction/

Do not be the person who has three conversations at once. Do not be the friend who speaks, but looks elsewhere. Just be where you are, and you will command that the other person be with you in that moment, as well.

3. *Love the mundane.*
Maximizing time is just like any habit. Pilates, Tai Chi and yoga are powerful forms of physical fitness because they allow you to practice being present in your coming 24 hours. Anything that allows you to form small habits builds discipline. You need to be disciplined about how you spend your time. Every morning I follow a consistent routine that may seem mundane to others, but it helps me make my commitments on a large scale. I will always have my large water bottle, I will always have a protein shake, I always have my time for prayer and reflection, and I always choose good ingredients for my daughter's lunch. I always make it a goal to be present and positive with my family at breakfast. Once I check all the boxes for these basic daily routine items, I know I have started my day with an attitude of discipline for maximizing my time. Routines provide you with skills to take pride in the insignificant, so you can value the amazing feeling and are humble when the significant comes. Of course, when you are a present person, you realize there are no insignificant moments.

ENERGY

To be able to maximize your day, you need to build your energy source. You knew this part of the book was coming, right? A powerful person has three parts: soul, heart, and body. I cannot stress enough the importance of taking care of your health to find your power and purpose.

To be powerful for my children and myself is exactly why I embarked on a journey to make physical fitness a pathway to my extraordinary. From what I put in my body (greens, fruits, water and produce that give me energy), to little changes like parking at the end of a parking lot so I get a brisk walk in every day, I focus on letting my body tap into its energy resources.

Once I established my foundational routine, I kicked it up a notch. Yes, in my busiest times I became more physical because it helped me be more productive as a mother, wife and professional.

I started doing triathlons five years ago and have not stopped. I share this to show you that anyone can maximize his or her potential in all areas of life by using the tool of great physical fitness. It is not for vanity, nor for a dress size, but it is for the energy you need to be your version of magnificent.

It is like life. You go through different stages and different challenges. You think you are prepared and you know how it will feel, but you have no idea. You do not have to win; you just have to cross the finish line smiling.

I have met many women who have impressed me in different capacities. Women are exceptionally strong beings. After all, they bear children. What bigger sign of physical and mental strength is there? Unfortunately, I have also met women who are facing difficult challenges and sometimes forget their strength. They forget they have the capacity to face anything and come out victorious while immersed in the most difficult situations.

This amnesia of sorts doesn't only happen to women facing difficult situations, but also to women who are facing daily, tiring routines. All the errands, family responsibilities, and professional and personal obligations can make any woman feel that she has nothing left to give. But this is when physical fitness is so important.

Are you an athlete? For anyone who has been playing sports and competing all her life, this is a simple question to answer. For someone who had knots in her stomach during gym class and anxiety when she was timed for her fastest mile in junior high, the question is probably also easy to answer, with a resounding "No."

Well, I am going to challenge you. I am going to ask you to let go of your past labels here. The definition of an athlete is "a person possessing the natural or acquired traits, such as strength, agility, and endurance, which are necessary for physical exercise or sports, especially those performed in competitive contexts."

What if you were never given an opportunity to explore your natural traits? Perhaps your parents sent you straight to the chess and debate clubs. Or your parents never experienced the joy of physical activity themselves. All these factors could have designed your personal experiences for you to believe that you are not an athlete, when in reality, maybe you always have been one. You are a living, breathing daughter, wife, mother or grandmother running around for your family. You are jumping through obstacle courses and bouncy houses for your kids, and developing great guns in your forearms as you carry your baby and cook at the same time. Have you ever considered seeing yourself as a pretty good athlete?

I'd been running track since I was 12. It had always been one of my passions, but swimming and biking were not a given for me. My swimming experience basically consisted of hanging out with my friends at the pool and doing what I needed to do to pass with a 'satisfactory' in gym class. Biking was even worse. I had not been on a bike since I was ten.

Even athletes have fears and limitations. I played rugby in college and surfed off the coast of Costa Rica. Yes, I could tackle someone without fear and could work a surfboard (which I used to lean on to not drown) and a paddleboard, but I could not make a bike move.

I needed to learn how to swim and bike correctly to be able to finish a triathlon. I made the decision to complete a summer triathlon and train for it at my gym. I confessed my aspiration to my trainer. I also told her I could not swim or bike; I just wanted to go for it. The race was in June, and it was already mid-April. You can imagine the look on her face. I was asking for a crash course. But because I believed in me, she believed in me.

She taught me to swim and helped me during my first swim in a lake. She taught me bike mechanics and took me on long bike rides. It was challenging, but I got through it. My first race, I surprised my family by having their names on my shirt. The second race, I crossed the finish line with my daughter in my arms for the last 20 meters. These are memories that will last a lifetime and I honestly felt like a superhero.

I reminded myself of my physical strength—of my resilience as a mother, wife, daughter, sister, and as a woman. If all women carried the knowledge of their own limitless strength, imagine what else they could accomplish.

If you do not have the energy even to implement a strategy to create more, start small. Triathlons may not be for you, but steady, small commitments to maintaining energy or physical fitness are necessary and completely doable for every human being. You can begin with a short walk every day or a yoga class, or even a simple game of chase with your children. If it yields energy, participate and make using this tool a priority as a daily practice.

REST FOR A REDO

This tool is simple. You need to shut down at the end of the day. Shut off your phone and pick a decent time to go to sleep. Your body needs to rest for the amazing things you will do each next day.

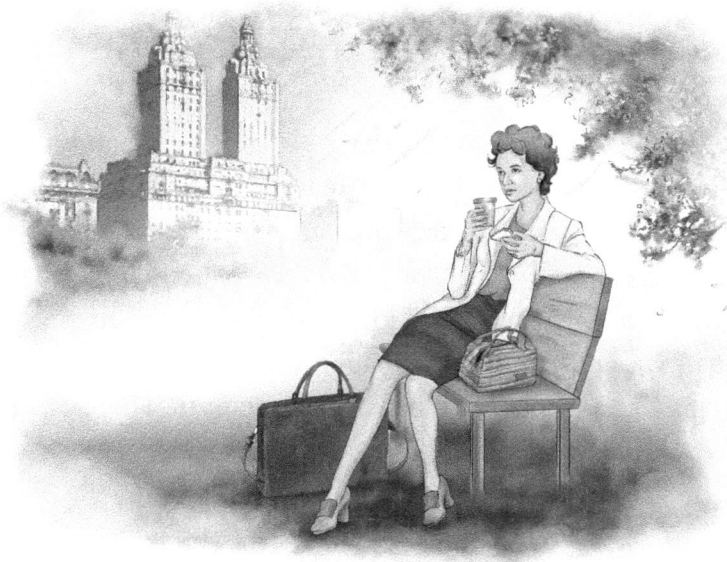

Chapter 9

PURPOSE

Your Purpose Changes with Your Life Seasons

It is so important to know what our values are and that a higher power is guiding us. We have different seasons in our lives, such as college, entering the workforce, being married or remaining single, becoming a parent; these all require us to show up mentally and physically.

You Do Not Just Have One Purpose in Life

Many people will search their entire lives, break off relationships, quit jobs and leave things unfinished because they feel their present circumstances are dragging them away from their purpose. This quest is filled with heartbreak, disappointment, and frustration. Having one purpose in life is having one experience to summarize our whole person. This could not be further from reality.

Working with Your Purpose

We are dynamic beings with a multitude of experiences, emotions and seasons in life; thus we play many roles. I do not see any single goal as the purpose of a lifetime; I see it as part of the pulse of life. Your purpose and your living existence have an interdependent relationship: they need each other to thrive. One does not guide the other. But for this to happen, you need to give your living existence respect for its autonomy.

Let me elaborate in simpler terms. When people are working toward one goal, they are focused on one aspect of their whole being. For some people, it's money, a certain political title, an Oscar or a family. If they do not meet their goal, they feel like failures for not finding their destiny. If they do achieve their goal, they may feel unfulfilled, realizing that the purpose was only a small part of a larger picture.

I recently read the story of super-power Ronda Rousey. She was celebrated as the ultimate undefeated UFC female fighter. Movies, marketing campaigns, and large sponsorships were all at her fingertips. She was considered a heroine. People saw her as the new feminist icon.

Rousey saw her purpose as being a fighter…until she faced the inevitable, when she lost miserably to Holly Holm at UFC 193. Rousey confessed openly the difficulties she had in finding herself after the defeat, saying she fell into a deep depression regarding what her role in the world was supposed to be after the defeat. She said she was so committed to following what her purpose was that it impacted how she did in the fight itself. She would share in an interview after the defeat of continuing to fight even after she was badly injured: "I kept saying to myself, 'You're OK, keep fighting. You're OK, keep fighting'…I just feel so embarrassed. How I fought after that is such an embarrassing representation of myself."

This is an example of when adults feel that their one goal is their ultimate purpose and when circumstances fail them, they feel lost.

Another example of someone who was driven by what they feel is their God-given purpose can be found the world of politics. Senator John Edwards, a distinguished attorney, spent his whole life building a political career, to run for the most powerful position in the world. He was known as the down-to-earth, humble, hardworking family man who was a great shot for the Democratic presidential candidate.

In the midst of his election run, Edwards was cheating on his wife who was on his campaign trail, supporting him even though she was diagnosed with an aggressive form of cancer. Elizabeth Edwards was ill, and she and John had suffered the loss of their son years earlier, making it seem their marital bond was unbreakable. He cheated on his wife, and fathered a child, and then used campaign funds to hide the child and keep the scandal at bay.

John Edwards stated: "Can I explain to you what happened?....Ego. Self-focus, self-importance. I was slapped down to the ground when my son,

Wade, died in April of 1996. But then after that, I got elected to the Senate…becoming a national public figure. All of which fed a self-focus, egotism, a narcissism that leads you to believe that you can do whatever you want. You're invincible. And there will be no consequences. And nothing, nothing could be further from the truth."

Both of these people lived to fulfill their goals, which they thought was their purpose. They put everything they had toward one goal to the detriment of their bodies, their relationships or their personal values.

A Fork in the Road: Universal Dilemma

There are forks in the road of life. Do we get married, or do we move to City X and take the new job and delay the marriage until later? Do we start a family or wait until we have all our finances in order, despite the fact that we are getting older? Do we take a corporate job that pays well or do we work for a nonprofit and help the less fortunate for the next three years?

If you have always believed that you have only one purpose in life, your personal narrative could make decisions very difficult. After you make choices, you will always be suffering from buyers' remorse when things get tough, as they often do.

Let me share with you a notion that will change your life. It's an undeniable truth that if you internalize, will help you always make the best decisions to fulfill your purpose at any given time.

Your life is a set of experiences, and your purpose is to live in those experiences that serve you, using your spiritual guide as your compass.

This statement brings together the building blocks that we have been discussing thus far:

- Building a cocoon to learn about your values
- Staying true to your values
- Believing that there is a spiritual compass
- Being present to hear what your SL is telling you

Once you realize that your life is a dynamic set of experiences, you will never be perplexed when choosing a path. You will realize that a certain path might not be good for you now, but you may revisit it later. You will know if a certain scenario is right for you because your spiritual compass is guiding you. It will come into your life again when the circumstances are not so crowded. You will know that when you are embracing a certain event in your life, you are not saying goodbye to another forever. All events and people that come into your life are deliberate, and they are here to serve you. They are here to help you serve your current purpose with full intensity and impact right now.

You might be asking: *My spiritual compass is guiding me, but it is tugging me in two directions. How do I know which one is correct?* Well, there is a trick for that, as well.

Knowing Your Non-negotiables

When I had my children, I never wanted them to feel that they were second to anything else on my list, especially when they were young. I knew, based on how my parents made me feel, that self-assurance starts at home. If you feel that you are the most valued person on earth to someone, you will always value yourself and in turn value others.

I always wanted my parents to know I was grateful to them, that I valued their sacrifices and love. Also, that their effort should make them proud and result in something that provided them comfort. I want to stay healthy, as much as I can control my health. I want to maximize the time I have here and be filled with energy so I can be an example to my children. Lastly, I wanted to live a life that was in accordance with my faith. These four things were my non-negotiables:

- Caring for my kids
- Making my parents proud
- Living a healthy lifestyle
- Upholding the tenets of my faith.

These were things in life that I would not ever want to give up no matter what incredible opportunity came my way. No matter the exciting possibility, if it took me away from my non-negotiables, I would walk away. These non-negotiables and my values always help me make decisions whenever I am at a fork in the road. And if you are living entirely in a dynamic way, there will be plenty.

Passion and Joy = Non-negotiables

If you are wondering what your non-negotiables are, they are the people or things that would break your heart if they were no longer present in your life. The key is being honest about who and what you absolutely cannot live without, and committing to them. These people and things are always connected to joy and passion. They could be your family, your love of being creative, your dedication to social justice or your simple commitment to

> " *I think you can be a dreamer, but you should also include a dose of reality.* "
>
> *Mariam Sobh*

authenticity. They are the things that keep you alive, that make you feel like everything in your life, when you are in close proximity to such things, activities or people, make you excited for each next day. If you always keep your passion and joy a priority and stay true to your values, no matter what path you take at forks in the road, you will fulfill the purpose that brings you the most satisfaction.

How to Follow Your Current Purpose

Let's say you have chosen a path, a purpose for this season in your life. It could be a personal or professional purpose. How do you fulfill it? Many believe that once you are in the zone of fulfilling your purpose, things all of a sudden become smooth. There are no bumps in the road, and you are supposed to go about your business and get busy, and all will fall into place. Nothing could be further from the truth! Yes, there will be contentment in what you are doing, ease in your soul, but there will still be a struggle in its execution.

Mariam Sobh is a journalist, entrepreneur, and actress who has performed in the Conservatory at the acclaimed Second City Training Center in Chicago. Here is what she had to say on the subject: "I think you can be a dreamer, but you should also include a dose of reality. What I wish I had done was stop worrying and obsessing over getting into television right away. I didn't see that there are so many other paths that could lead to that ultimate goal. I also didn't realize that sometimes these are life lessons and maybe it's not my time right now to be in television."

If you want to achieve a goal that other people think is unattainable, try a unique route—figure out a way to possibly get you there that no one else is attempting. And finally, never listen to naysayers. It's easier said than done, but many times people say things negatively because they wish they were able to do what you're doing and aren't able to voice those feelings appropriately.

Have you ever felt when you set out to do something you desire that there are plenty of obstacles in your way? We have all experienced this before. When we encounter such a situation, we have two choices: give up or keep going. If we choose to give up, then we have let go of a goal. If we keep going, we have chosen to fulfill our purpose.

In the *Last Lecture* by Dr. Randy Pausch, he says that obstacles are not there to halt you from reaching your goal, but to help you see how badly you want it. I could not agree with this more. For me, it goes even deeper.

Obstacles I experience when I am in the process of fulfilling my purpose, in my opinion, are just tests from God. They are tests that give me an opportunity to show God that I want something, and I believe with His help and guidance I will keep pushing in the hopes that my efforts will reward me with the fulfillment of a goal.

Get ready for bumps in the road as you travel your chosen path. Know they are only there to teach you the undeniable truth: nothing worth doing boldly is a cakewalk, and that is why you were chosen for the journey.

Failure: Learn to Embrace It for Your Purpose

I knew I wanted to be a lawyer ever since I was in grade school. I loved the law. During law school, I was invited to a program in Switzerland with dignitaries and politicians to learn about law and international relations. When I graduated from law school, I enjoyed defending others who could not defend themselves. I took the law seriously. So, imagine how incredible it was for someone like me, to actually fail the bar exam.

I was devastated. I didn't understand how someone who understood the complexities of the law could fall so short. Others who were far less impassioned or knowledgeable about the law passed the exam easily. I soon realized that it was the type of multiple-choice test that I could not take easily.

I tried again and studied for the incredibly demanding two-day exam. I failed again. Now the whispers and hushes started among my peers. But that did not stop me. I tried again and failed. I had failed five times and had reached a fork in the road. Giving up was not an option. Now, many wise people would say I should have seen it as a sign from the universe that I was not supposed to be doing this. But I knew my purpose at that time in my life and that I had to do what needed to be done. I understood it deeply. My purpose was to become a lawyer. I had done so much preparation for it; I had such a passion for it, and I saw myself as an attorney.

For me, the fork in the road was whether I should try something completely out of the box or try this exam the same way one more time? I decided the former, because the law gave me joy and passion. I called the president of the Bar of Admissions at his office number.

I left him numerous messages until he finally responded to me. I told him on the phone, "I would like to drive three hours to come and see you. I want you to see someone who has failed five times and what they look like." Of course, he was taken back by the conversation. He told me he was very busy, but did feel bad. I then asked him if I could send him an email. He agreed. I wrote him a long, detailed letter listing all my accomplishments, my legal policy work and advocacy, and my pro bono assistance to other lawyers.

In a nutshell, I was begging and pleading for the board to make an exception. One week went by, and then two weeks went by. No response. So I decided to contact him again.

I was sitting by myself at a brunch place, and I dialed his number. I did not know if he would even pick up at this point. He did. I told him that I had sent him a long letter and I had not heard back. He said the following: "I was so inspired by your letter. You have done such great work. The board met, and the whole board got a copy of your letter. We were all inspired, but our hands are tied. You have to take the exam again. We all need you to take it again." A lump formed in my throat, but his words made an impact on me. It reassured me that my work was valuable and that even the president of the board that administers this exam does not want me to give up. This only reassured me of my purpose at that time, to take the exam. I took it again, a sixth time, and I passed.

My father once remarked while we were driving in the car after one of my failed attempts, "Once you fail enough but you keep trying, that attribute becomes a part of who you are, it becomes your personality." I internalized those words. Failure taught me that I was a persistent person; it defined my character as someone who has an unconquerable will. When I look back at my childhood years, I realized that I had been this person all along. I used to study long into the night, trying to understand simple math concepts that seemed foreign to me. I would run for hours, trying to beat a certain time for an upcoming track meet. I was always pushing for things.

A 800-pound gorilla takes different forms for each one of us. If you are consistent in the way you respond to those gorillas, they simply become a charted territory with different names, and sometimes, with higher stakes. Such was the case when I was trying to become a mother. I would see many young women having babies, conceiving with ease. They would complain about how much work it was and how little sleep they got. They even discussed how they could not deal with more children. Little did they know that I was struggling to become pregnant. How I would have loved to be bothered at night by a crying baby, or have an aching body caused by carrying my little miracle. I longed for the chance to become a mother.

My husband and I were facing unexplained infertility, a painful, emotional reality that many people experience today. We went through medical treatments, including countless shots, and blood tests, with constant negative results. We were told that becoming parents might never be a reality for us. Being told something would never happen and that a certain experience was not meant for me was a familiar obstacle. Yet I knew that at that point in my life, my purpose was to become a mother.

I put all my effort into becoming a mother: I tried new procedures, I prayed, I asked other people to pray, and I tried holistic treatments. I tried everything I could get my hands on to fulfill my purpose at that time. I am now, by God's divine will, a mother of three. Yes, persistence is in my character, failure is my catalyst, and my will is my armor.

To fulfill your purpose, you must accept failing at something and get comfortable with the word failure itself. Failure is a gift that brings you one step closer to your solutions. Competition can energize you and push you to stay ahead of the game. Competition keeps you creative. Once you recognize these assets, you will never fear or try to avoid them.

Experts: There Are None

When you are planning to execute a goal, and you are deep in the planning stages, filled with details and deadlines, you might get those little internal whispers like:

> "You can't do it."
> "You are not meant for it."
> "You don't know enough."

These thoughts that cross your mind are sometimes powerful enough to dissuade you, to convince you that you are not worthy. I have met many intelligent, amazing people who have much stronger skills than mine in so many areas, and whose intellect I admire. I always wondered why they never accomplished more. Why were they not pursuing all the things I could see them excel at? Sometimes I'd get a response to such inquiries: "That is just not what I wanted to do," or "This thing X interested me more."

These responses I understood. However, it hurt when I heard things like, "I could never tackle something that complex," or "I don't know how to do that." It bothered me because I knew: (1) they did not truly see themselves and (2) at some point in their life, the "Expert Fraud" got to them. Somebody convinced them that they were not enough.

If there is one thing that failing five times has taught me, it is that there are no experts. Nobody knows everything. Everyone can learn something new to add to his or her knowledge base. Once you realize that everybody is a work in progress, you become aware that not knowing enough is part of your journey to knowing more. Put another way: you learn from your ignorance what you actually need to learn.

I clerked for a very prestigious law clinic out of law school, one of the many things I did as I studied for the bar exam. I once crafted a legal memo and turned it in to my superior. I was very proud of it and could not wait to share it. My superior thought the format, the set-up, and the analysis were off the mark. She did not agree with any of my assessments, and though she was trying to be polite, she just did not align with anything I had written. I did not agree with her, and I also knew my disagreement had no value. This was a feeling I had experienced before and I would experience again, that someone who is "in the know" would believe and make me feel that I did not know I what I was doing. The key was to reflect on what she was saying and put myself in a position of learning.

In that instance and ever since, I have tried to react the same way, and it has helped me grow. I would not become defiant in my ways and ignore critique. Rather, I would take the critique and discover how I could improve. What helps me is that I do not see others as experts. I see them as people who know more than I do right now. They probably knew just as much as I did (or less) in the past. This would help me gain perspective on feedback from someone more knowledgeable.

Instead of focusing on the negative feelings and my bruised ego, I would learn from a peer. This was not a peer who knew everything, but someone who was little more ahead of me in the game. I also reminded myself that negative feelings, not-so-bright moments, and failures are things that all people of all levels feel. Being told by someone you do not belong–and you believing them–is the fastest way for you to be derailed from your current purpose. Instead, understand it is their purpose at this moment to challenge you. Take the challenge and make your path toward your current destiny.

Competition and Ego: How They Can Misguide You

Now, let's be honest. You can be very in tune with your SL and really be focused on what you are tirelessly doing to fulfill your purpose; then the universe will throw you a curveball. This curveball will agitate your sense of direction. It will have you doubt yourself and your place in this world and try to convince you that you are off course. When that happens, be prepared for it and learn how to squash it so it does not distract you. Recognize whether the curveball is a hint that you really are off course, or just a manifestation of your insecurity that is making you doubtful. Let me illustrate an example. For the past five years, you have been creating a business online for women who need direction on craft-making. You have been busy finding content and building relationships. Though the progress has been slow, it has been rewarding. You love the emails you get from women who have gained joy from your website. Here come the curveballs:

Scenario 1:

You attend an unrelated seminar and sit next to someone looking for an expert in craft-making content. It surprises you. What are the chances? She tells you she runs a popular website with huge amount of followers and the only thing missing is a DIY section on crafts. She is intrigued with your work and gives you her contact info. You meet with her a couple of times.

You have a new opportunity, to wrap up your own sole proprietorship and join this massive company that is giving you a great audience and quadrupling your followers. You will make more money, have more exposure, and gain direction from peers who are already succeeding at an online business. But you will no longer be self-employed.

No matter how you look at it, learning of this opportunity is a curveball in the perfect five-year plan you had for your business. You consider that maybe you were not meant to be the CEO of a company but rather a collaborator in a bigger pool with exponential growth. You are filled with excitement and hope. The energy you feel is positive.

Scenario 2:
You are watching the *Today Show* and see an interview of a woman who has just started an online craft-making company. And guess what: it is very similar to yours. Except, her company works with mothers of little girls. Her company is hitting it out of the ballpark after the *Today Show*. You see her on *Good Morning America*, and local news shows. Your brain starts doing flips while your stomach gets unusual knots. You start thinking, *Is this a sign? Perhaps I am not supposed to be doing this. Clearly I was meant to see this show to realize I have been doing this all wrong.*

Immediately you pull out a sketchpad, and you start scribbling ideas for how you can make your company more like the one you saw on TV. The more you write, the more anxious you feel. You become obsessed with this competitor. You search how their website runs and the background of the founder, and you start comparing your journey to hers. Anxiety leads you to feel insecure, filling your head with negative, destructive thoughts such as: "I am just not good at this," "I can't succeed at anything," or "Things come so easily to other people." now you are not only trying to create something different, but you are distracted from what you were originally doing, as well.

Now, let's examine the first scenario. Something unexpected happens. You are excited about this new development. You are assessing your options. The new curveball makes you feel good about yourself and your work.

Regardless of what you decide, you know that you are doing something positive for somebody and putting something worthy of marvel in the universe. You want to create more, learn more and take more chances. Contrast it to the second scenario. Something unexpected happens. You are left feeling anxious about the development. You are not only assessing options, you are assessing yourself. The new curveball makes you feel negatively about yourself and your abilities. Regardless of how you decide to move forward, you are left feeling that you are off-target, not on the radar, and just unnecessary. You want to find shortcuts, seek validation or ultimately if your body and mind tell you to, quit.

I do not have to lay out for you which scenario is a helpful hint vs. which one is an insecurity-inducing distraction. Clearly the second example has the potential to take you off-course. The key indicators are all the negative feelings of hopelessness, self-doubt and self-hate—feelings that ultimately lead to short-term and long-term inertia.

In contrast, things that are supposed to be a sign should give you peace, move you forward in some way. You may start reassessing where you are and your next move, but you do not start reassessing your abilities or your intelligence. Even if it is a hint that makes you feel uncomfortable (like that your significant other is being unfaithful), you are grateful quite quickly that you are discovering some truth in your benefit.

Now that you have recognized the distraction that is not serving as a sign of what you should do next, you have to learn how to make the curveball work for you. How do you frame the discovery you made on the *Today Show* as a positive reinforcement for you, or in the alternative, squash it? First of all, you have to understand that all information coming to you can be placed in a category by you. Either place it in a mental trash can as soon as you realize it is making you anxious, or see it as an asset by assigning it positive assessment words. Both options will automatically take the negativity out of the situation.

In this second scenario, you will say, "People really love crafts. Look at how well this is being received by the national media! Look how great this woman is doing. Just reminds me that so many people enjoy what I am doing, as well! Maybe I can interview her and include her on my site." This way of assessing information reminds you that everything that crosses your path has the ability to serve you if you have the correct intention of contributing something positive in the universe, either through your talent, your work or your time. Adopt the habit of viewing everything from a vantage point of positivity. It gives you moments of clarity and inspiration, such as inviting the other woman illustrated in the second scenario for an interview. Collaboration vs. competition always takes you farther.

Reliance on Praise for Direction

Social media feedback can mislead you into believing you have the cutest baby in the world or that you are the most stylish person in your office. The same goes for praise on your purpose.

Accept compliments with a nice thank-you, a nod to someone taking the time to praise you. But praise that elevates your ego beyond reasonable levels of humility is quite different. There is an important distinction to understand: Praise as an indication of Purpose vs. Praise as an indication of Appreciation.

In the first case, you are taking cues from others people's assessment of you to determine your next moves. This is problematic because it completely negates your responsibility in doing the hard work of figuring out your purpose at a given time. It places the burden on the praise-giver, who only knows a little about you and not your whole person or current circumstances. Even if the praise is given to you for a certain talent you have from someone who knows you really well, that is just a part of you. Here are some examples of praise that could misdirect your intentions:

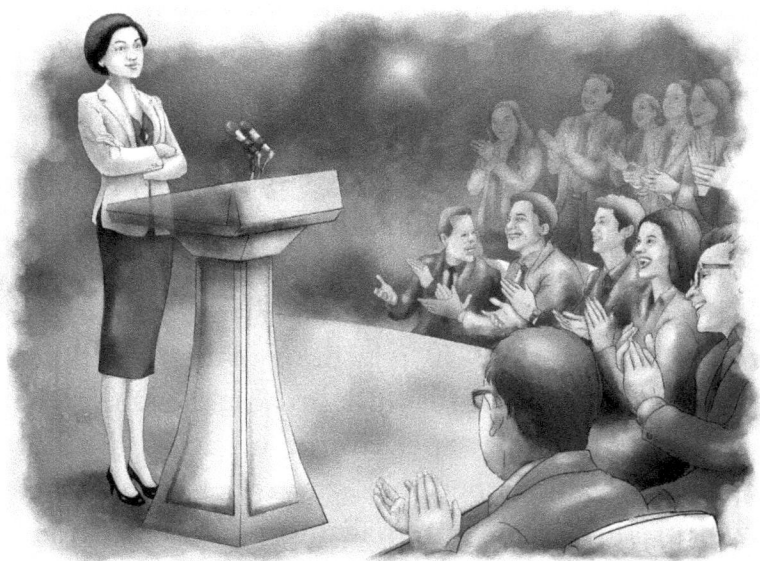

"You have such a beautiful voice.
You should sing for a living!"

"You are a great organizer.
You are meant to be an executive director."

"You are so charismatic that
you should be a public speaker."

These are all nice compliments, but they should be seen as flattering, and not indicators of your purpose. They are just recognition of one part of you. Your real indications come from your inner core. When you are on the right track to fulfilling your purpose, your feet are grounded on the floor so strongly it does not matter what positive or negative statements you hear.

By contrast, when your ego is looking for praise to determine your direction, to fuel you, instead of your own passion, you're going to be left unfulfilled. J. K. Rowling, the author of the *Harry Potter* series, received more than 30 rejections of her book, yet she still kept moving forward, because she knew that publishers' opinions, positive or negative, did not define the value of her book. It was her belief in her own product itself. Internalizing praise or critique correctly is an art and takes practice. Remember the story of Senator Edwards? Yes, somebody told him he should be president.

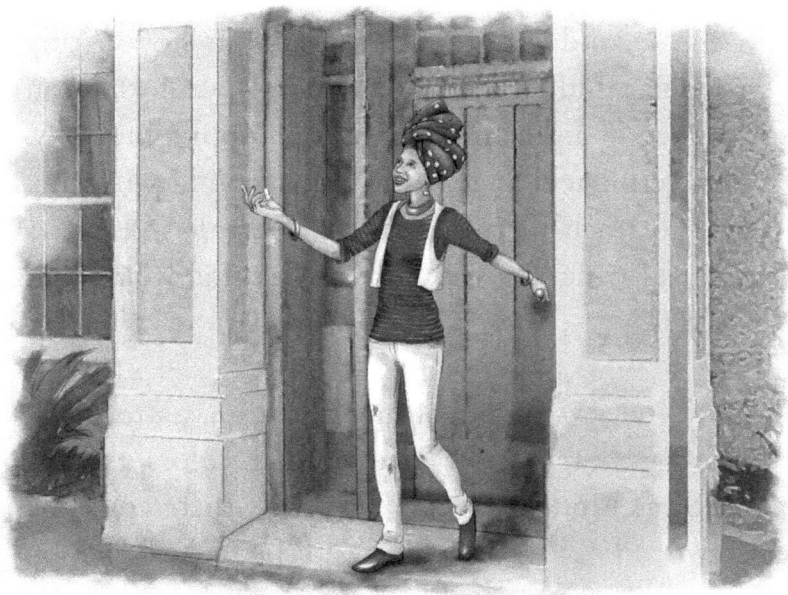

Chapter 10

YOUR JOURNEY LEADS YOU
TO A BIGGER WORLD

Your Presence Is Deliberate

I have written this book at a point in the history of this world when the women of communities, states, and nations are needed more than ever as powerful beings fulfilling their destinies.

In the second chapter, I spoke about how a tiny caterpillar undergoes major physical transformation in a cocoon and comes out as a blooming butterfly. The caterpillar changes and no doubt suffers growing pains to reach its full capacity. When it spreads its beautiful wings, it soars into the natural world that awaits it.

Have you ever studied the intricate patterns of butterfly wings—how many vivid colors, shapes and dimensions there are? It seems there could be no two alike. It is difficult to not be mesmerized by their display of beauty, the way they flicker, float and dance from one flower to another.

This is also you: a beautiful miracle of gifts bursting with potential that the world is just waiting for you to share. I wrote this book for you, for me and for all of us. I wrote it because in the end, we are givers. We are all intermediaries of sorts. We're messengers who bring the gifts of the divine to their rightful owners.

It's for these reasons that we need to answer the calling. We need to prepare by doing the necessary work of empowering ourselves. It is our duty to come to task.

We Are All Connected

All of us have some real, practical obstacles facing us that add additional challenges to each of our paths of empowerment. Women around the world have financial challenges, physical challenges and cultural and emotional baggage that we carry on a daily basis. We all can cite a laundry list of items that continue to hold us down, disempower us and make us feel us small, yet we have a hard time giving recognition to each other's laundry lists. We often don't validate others' experiences and struggles. I stress this because the road to personal strength has to incorporate the ability to support others, whose experiences differ from yours, and the ability to be humbled by others. In reality, we need each other.

Interdependence among women for the sake of the collective good impacts each woman as an individual. A community of support offers fresh perspectives and encouragement. Empathy, compassion and intuition bring us together rather than divide us. As you wish for your own personal growth and to find your voice, you have to support the voice of women who may oppose you. Changing the status quo does not happen in a vacuum. It is a collective reality. Hold your sister's hand and lift her up always.

We Are All Born as Royalty

I have traveled to many countries and have always been attracted to one thing in the people I meet: optimism. I have seen women in poverty who have the graciousness of a queen, leaving me humbled. Optimism, I believe, is the true heart of royalty, and royalty is a state of being that makes you understand your own wealth, its power and your responsibility to pay it forward.

In an interview, Princess Diana was asked if she believed she would live to be Queen of England. "I want to be the queen of people's hearts. But I do not believe that I will be the queen of this country, because the establishment does not want me to be queen. They consider me a nonstarter. Because I work with my heart not my head and I do not play with the rules. I know it has gotten me in trouble sometimes. But somebody has got to love those people and show it."

When questioned as to why the establishment at the time did not like her individuality, she responded, "I think strong women have dealt with this throughout history. *Where does she get this strength? What will she do with it? Where will she go with it?*"

Princess Diana died at the age of 36 before she ever became Queen of England, but she did die as the Queen of Hearts. We do not choose where we are born or what family we are born into, but we can all still have immense impact, no matter what our resources. We are able to choose the kind of world we build for ourselves.

> *Only you can decide what is right for you and when. There is no right answer outside of you.*
>
> Eileen Donahoe

You Are a Visionary

Eileen Donahoe, the Global Affairs Director of Human Rights Watch, holds a Masters, a JD and a PhD and has graduated from elite schools such as Harvard, Stanford, and Berekley. She also is a mother of four children. I asked her what she would tell women about taking leaps and chasing ambitions. She said, "To thine own self be true. Only you can decide what is right for you and when. There is no right answer outside of you. Each person is free to make his or her own choices and must live with those choices. But the important thing to remember is that if you can envision a path for yourself, it is possible to successfully follow that path, regardless of what others may tell you."

We all have the ability to become visionaries, to look beyond the distractions in front of us, to create an optimistic future that is better for ourselves and those around us. Visionaries lead movements. Movements are made up of individuals. Throughout history, we have seen impactful individuals who took it upon themselves to fight for the rights of others and themselves (women's rights, civil rights, workers' rights, children's rights).

Women are the foundations of every community, the teachers of each new generation. We have a great calling, requiring us to be focused, passionate and determined. Women can cause seismic changes to the status quo.

As you look through recent newsfeeds, you see genocide in the Middle East, hunger in Africa, police brutality on the streets of Chicago. You'll find suicides due to bullying, domestic violence and poverty in most American towns. You will see abandoned and sex-trafficked children all across the globe. Is this the world you want to raise your daughters to be queens of? More importantly, is this what you want for your world right now? Every day we make choices. We decide what to devote our energies to and how we choose to see the world around us. We can either fall into three categories:

- Fear–believing tragedies are inevitable.
- Apathy–accepting the status quo.
- Accountability–understanding our responsibility for our lives and the impact we can have others who are less fortunate.

The journey to personal power, the extraordinary belief that you are in the driver's seat of your circumstances, is only purposeful if you change others' lives for the better.

Be a Person of IMPACT: Execute Your Vision

If movements are made up of individuals, what traits do such trailblazers have in common? Look at Martin Luther King, Jr., Mahatma Gandhi, Mother

Teresa, Nelson Mandela, Malcolm X, Joan of Arc, and Abraham Lincoln. Whether it was creating discourse about injustice, using their hands to heal humanity or creating momentum toward changing systemic barriers for people, all these individuals did two valuable things that set them apart:

- They paid attention to the societal ills around them.

- They took ownership of becoming part of the solution.

All people of impact were ordinary people who understood the value of ordinary actions in extraordinary times.

Know Where You Are Most Needed

Not everyone can put on a backpack and travel the world to save the victims of atrocities. Being a person of impact does not mean a glamorous adventure of soul-searching and sacrifice that will land you on the cover of Time magazine. Impact looks different for everyone. It can be on the smallest scale of actions that have the biggest impact on one life, which in turn creates a domino effect for a community.

Be Good to Yourself

This is what my mother told me to do when facing any challenges or conflicts: "Be good to yourself." This meant that I should take care of my values with the highest level of integrity, so I can respect myself and nurture my character. We can all create a domino effect of positivity and possibility. But if we do not appreciate our own value, we will never understand the impact of our actions.

This book was a labor of love for me. I wanted to find a way to connect to those who were feeling lost in this world of superficiality and competition. I wanted to find a way to take you through a journey in which you realize that you are not here to compete. You are here to give, share, thrive and prosper.

I struggled with how to end this chapter—how to leave you with lasting words that remind you of your purpose and contributions to the world. After many edits, I came to the conclusion that perhaps the best way to end this book is to remind you of an undeniable truth–that there is a plan for you here.

There is a deliberate calling on your life and talents. A calling by the Creator that requires you to embrace your light, your shine and claim your place on this earth as significant. The world is waiting on you. I am waiting on you. We all need you. You are more than meets the eye, you always have been. You are more than pretty. You are powerful beyond your expectations.

" Each day is filled with opportunities to take steps towards your goals and interactions to help you brighten someone else's day. How are you uplifting others and your own goals today? Don't waste any moment you are given. It could be a defining moment for you. "

Maaria Mozaffar